100+
Baby Shower Games

by Joan Wai

author of 100+ Wedding Games

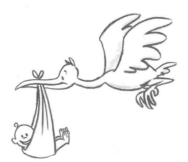

DISCLAIMER

The prospect of a baby is a happy and anxious time for new (and repeat) parents. Use your common sense and carefully evaluate the appropriateness of these games to the occasion and people attending. Though effort has been made to present these activities as a positive experience for players and spectators, fun and funny can be surprisingly subjective. The publisher and author disclaim any liability, physical or emotional, that may result from proper or improper use of the information herein.

A note about the cover:
Instructions for making a diaper cake like the one pictured on the cover can be found in the Baby Cakes game.

100+ Baby Shower Games
Copyright © 2005 by Joan Wai

ISBN: 0-9728354-1-5

Published in the U.S.A. by The Brainstorm Company, 11684 Ventura Blvd. #970, Studio City, CA 91604. www.TheBrainstormCompany.com

Cover and illustrations by Jun Falkenstein

Table of Contents

INTRODUCTION... 7

SPEED GAMES 9

    ARTISTIC SAVANT..9
    BEAN COUNTERS 10
    BLOWING KISSES...11
    BREAKFAST TIME...12
    BUNDLE UP 13
    CLOTHESHORSE CONTENTION 14
    DIDN'T MEAN TO BURST YOUR BUBBLE............15
    DOCTOR'S ORDERS......................................16
    DON'T WAKE THE BABY...............................18
    IN PLAIN SIGHT...19
    IT'S A WRAP 20
    MOBILE MOMMIES.....................................21
    PUTTING BABY TO BED 22
    QUADRUPLETS.. 23
    QUIET ENOUGH FOR A PIN DROP 24
    ROCK THE BABY.. 25
    RUSH DELIVERY 26
    SAFE TO EAT... 27
    SNIFFLES 28
    SPILT MILK 29
    SPOONING THE PUDDING......................... 30
    TYING THE CORD..31
    WEE GULPS... 32
    ZOO KEEPER.. 33

SIT DOWN GAMES... 35

    BABES IN TOYLAND 35
    BEDTIME STORY.. 36
    BELLY ACHE.. 37

BOTTOMS UP 38
CHAPERONE 39
CHILDPROOF 40
COST OF LIVING 41
COUNT OFF 42
CRIB SHEETS 43
CRY BABIES 44
DIAPER DUTY 45
HOUSEHOLD GOODS 46
LIL' MUGS 47
MOM'S PRIDE & JOY 48
MOMMY'S PURSE 50
RANDOM WINNER 51
SHOWER BAG 52
STATS 53
STORK DELIVERY 54
SWEET TALK 55
WHO'S YOUR MOMMA 56
WISDOM TEETH 57

MEMORY/WORD GAMES **59**

BABYING MOM 59
BABY SITTING 60
THE FAMILY NAME 61
THE FUNNIES 62
KIDDING AROUND 63
MATERNITY LEAVE 64
MEETING OF THE MINDS 65
MINDING YOUR FRUITS & VEGETABLES 66
MULTILINGUAL BABY 67
NAME CALLING 68
NEWS FLASH 69
OLD WIVES' TALES 70
PARTS OF A WHOLE 72
PETTING ZOO 73
PIECE OF CAKE 74

PINNED ON MOM...76
POPULARITY CONTEST.....................................77
RHYME AND REASON.......................................78
SWEET EXPECTATIONS.....................................79
TAKING NAMES...80
WE'RE IN THE MONEY.......................................81
WHISPERING SWEET NOTHINGS.......................82
WORD TO THE WISE..83

ACTIVE GAMES...85

BARNYARD CRITTERS.......................................85
COPYCAT...86
DATING..87
DIAPER SERVICE...88
DIAPER TAG..89
FEEDING TIME..90
FOOD GROUPS..91
GOOD NEIGHBORS..92
HANDYMAN..93
HEN PARTY...94
ICE CREAM SCOOPER..95
LENDING A HAND..96
LIKE TAKING CANDY FROM A BABY....................97
ONION PEELING..98
PACKING FOR THE HOSPITAL.............................99
PASS THE PACIFIER...100
PIN DOWN THE DUE DATE................................101
POP THE NEWS..102
PREGNANT PAUSE...103
SCRIBBLES...104
SOMETHING'S IN THE OVEN.............................105
STACK THE DECK...106
TOSS THE BOOTIE...107
UGLY DUCKLING...108
WATER WAIT...109

CRAFT GAMES **111**

BIB WEAR 111
BABY CAKES 112
BABY TALK 113
BOTTLE YOUR FEELINGS 114
CONCEIVING BABIES 115
IT'S ALL RELATIVE 116
KID'S PLAY 117
MATERNITY LINE 118
MOTHERHOOD MATTERS 119
MY BABY DOLL 120

APPENDIX **121**

SWADDLING A BABY 121
TAKING NAMES VARIATION 121
MORE FAMILY NAMES 122
WISDOM TEETH QUESTIONS 122
WHO'S YOUR MOMMA GAME SHEET 123
ONION PEELING VARIATION 124
PRODUCING A GREAT BABY STORY 125
PRIZE IDEAS 126

GAME INDEX **127**

INTRODUCTION

One of the things to expect when someone's expecting is a baby shower. This tradition of throwing a party to celebrate a woman eating for two is uniquely American. During her delicate condition, friends and family give baby gifts, enjoy some food with the bun in the oven, and play games in the family way.

No one quite knows how the modern baby shower came to be. History has a long tradition of people bestowing gifts on parents following a baby's birth. The baby shower as we know it today is the likely offspring of the bridal shower. The practice of filling a parasol with small gifts and opening it over the recipient's head to "shower" her with presents was first recorded in the 1890's. But since pregnant women stayed out of the public eye in the past, post-birth baby showers were the norm. Eventually someone must have gotten the idea that a pre-birth baby shower could provide some cheer to an expectant mother in her third trimester. This also allowed her friends to appreciate the physical changes unique to a woman carrying a child. Today, the mother's preference dictates whether to celebrate before or after the stork drops off its precious cargo.

No matter when the baby shower is held, a unique mix of people will attend. A co-worker, neighbor, sister, and former college roommate could all be meeting for the first time. Baby shower games are a fun and popular entertainment choice because of their broad appeal. These friendly competitions can also bridge a generation or language gap among attendees. Most importantly, organized activities take the pressure of entertaining off the pregnant guest of honor.

These parties have historically been for firstborns and attended by women only. But as the tradition continues to evolve, it now comes in the form of coed showers, adoption showers, and "a sprinkle" for the second (or more) baby.

A baby shower host should select games that mom is comfortable with and also enjoyable for the invitees to play. The type of games that appeal to a demure coed crowd may differ for a gathering of boisterous gals. With that in mind, games in this book are organized by the way they're played:

- ❏ **Speed Games**
  challenge a player's agility, speed, and/or coordination.
- ❏ **Sit Down Games**
  can be played sitting down.
- ❏ **Memory/Word Games**
  utilize memorization and/or word play.
- ❏ **Active Games**
  require some freedom of movement, but speed is not necessarily an advantage.
- ❏ **Craft Games**
  challenge the artist within and reward creativity.

The Game Index has game suggestions by occasion. In addition, your game selections can complement your party's theme.

Every game in this book can be played in under 10 minutes and is easily scalable to the number of participants. While most people attend a shower knowing games are a likely activity, there's no guarantee of 100% participation. Don't sweat it, these games are just as fun to observe as they are to play. If the majority of guests are veteran baby shower attendees, be sure to read the Variations/Tips for fresh and unique twists on classic crowd pleasers.

Awarding small prizes to players is not obligatory, but definitely facilitates enthusiastic participation. The Appendix has a list of economical prize suggestions. A gracious host should keep an eye out for a player who constantly comes in last during the games. Should the situation arise, lighten the mood by unexpectedly awarding a prize to the first and last place player while announcing that was a surprise of the game.

Encourage your guests to enjoy these giggle-inducing games with levity and good sportsmanship. A fun baby shower is a memorable baby shower.

SPEED GAMES

ARTISTIC SAVANT

Sketchy artists try to get the picture.

When
before/after baby is born

How
Give everybody who wants to play one crayon and large white paper plate. Tell people who choose to sit out (if any) that they will be called on to help with the second part of the game. Players set the plate on their head and sketch a teddy bear with the crayon onto their plate. The newborn artists have 30 seconds to show off their quick draw.

When time's up, sketchers hold their drawing in front of them. Any guests who sat out now get to draw a bead on the best rendition of a teddy bear.

Variation/Tips
☐ If everybody decides to play together, have the group vote on their favorites or simply celebrate each picture's uniqueness.
☐ Want to keep playing? Go another round and select something else to draw. Possible subjects: a baby, stroller, crib, bottle, portrait of mom, etc.
☐ If drawing on one's head is too physically demanding, let players draw on the plate in front of them. The only stipulation is that they may not lift their crayon from the plate once they start drawing!
☐ See who's quickest on the draw by shortening the time limit to 10 seconds!
☐ Instead of having guests vote for their favorite, let mom select the winner.

BEAN COUNTERS

A sorting game that's full of beans.

When
before/after baby is born

How
Select three people to play. Pour two tablespoons each of the following dried beans into a bowl for each player: black-eyed beans, kidney beans, and pinto beans. Sit players in front of each bowl. Spill the beans to players that they have to be the first to pull out all the kidney beans from their bowl. Easy, right? Well, they have to do it blindfolded!

Give your bean counters one minute to complete their tasks, then remove their blindfolds for the results. For each non-kidney bean they've pulled out, if any, they have to put one kidney bean back in the bowl as penalty. Non-kidney beans don't count toward the total. Whoever amounts to the biggest hill of kidney beans in the end is your bean sorting champion.

Variation/Tips
❑ To make this bean poll easier to play, don't use blindfolds and have players sort out all three beans into separate piles. Remove the time limit and just have them race against one another.
❑ This alternative is more fun for a group. Pour two pounds each of the three different dried legumes into a baby tub (or large pail) and have as many players who can crowd around the tub play at once. Give each sorter a paper cup to hold their collection. Whoever can collect the most of a specific bean of their choosing in 30 seconds wins.
❑ Another alternative: pour a pound of dry oatmeal into a bowl and stir in a generous handful of paperclips. Have players take turns trying to sort out as many paperclips as they can in 20 seconds with their eyes closed.

BLOWING KISSES

A blow by blow kissing competition.

When
before/after baby is born

How
The goal is to blow a kiss across a room first. You'll need two ping pong balls and two plastic bulb syringes. Imprint a lipstick stained kiss on each ping pong ball—these are your kisses. In a wide hallway or open room, create a start line with masking tape, then mark a finish line 9 feet away (about one and a half body-lengths long). Select pairs of players to compete against each other.

Give each Joe Blow a kiss (the ball) and a syringe. At the word "go," players blow their kiss forward by squeezing the syringe over and over to puff air onto the ball. Whoever blows their kiss over the finish line first can kiss and make-up with their rival afterwards.

Variation/Tips
❑ Spray shellac onto the ball to prevent the lip print from staining your playing surface. Or, tape some clear tape over the kiss.

❑ You can play ball just about anywhere, on the carpet (if it's not too plush) or linoleum or cement; different surfaces provide different challenges.

❑ Have players go one at a time to see who can blow their kiss the farthest on one squeeze.

❑ No bulb syringe is needed for this variation. Set a kiss on the edge of a table. A blindfolded player stands in front of their kiss, facing the table. At the word "go," the player takes five steps backwards (away from the table), turns around in place two times, then takes five steps forwards to return to the table. Using their mouth, player tries to blow their kiss as far as possible with one breath. (Some players may miss completely.)

Fast and furious flapjack flipping fun.

When
before/after baby is born

How
You'll need two spatulas, oven mitts, and dinner plates. Make eight "pancakes" by cutting eight plate-sized rounds out of quilt batting.

Select two players to compete against each other in this flapjack flipping face off. Give each flipper one spatula to hold, one oven mitt to wear on their other hand, and one dinner plate to hold with the gloved hand.

Lay out four pancakes on a kitchen counter for each person. Blindfold your short-order cooks and position them in front of their flapjacks. (Space the players an arm-length apart.) The two have one minute to use the spatula to flip their pancakes, one at a time, from the grill (the counter) to their plate.

What makes this fun is that the pancakes are so light, your dueling chefs are never quite sure if they've even got a pancake on their spatula, much less flipped it onto the plate! The person who serves up the most pancakes onto their plate can flip out over their victory.

Variation/Tips
- If neither player dishes up any pancakes in time, declare a tie. Give them the option of a rematch or give other players a go.
- This is one of those games where it's just as fun to be a spectator as it is to be a participant.

BUNDLE UP

Sock monkeys lay it on thick to win.

When
before/after baby is born

How
Materials needed to play: a pair of thick gloves and at least ten pairs of old socks. Your footloose players remove their shoes, but keep their socks on. Taking turns, a foot soldier first has to wear the gloves (on their hands), then tries to pull on as many socks on one foot as they can in one minute. Record the number of socks your sock jockey is able to get on, then let the next trooper sock to it.

Treat this game of footsie with kid gloves because you'll need to put your best foot forward and sock away the most footwear to win!

Variation/Tips
❑ Go to a thrift store to look for a variety of cheap socks. Or buy a couple of inexpensive multi-packs.
❑ Get a large quantity of old socks to make this into a group game. Seat players on the floor in a circle and dump all the socks in the center. See how many socks they can pull on in one minute. Player with most layers on wins.
❑ Blindfold three volunteers and make them all wear a pair of thick gloves. Hand each player a pair of large pantyhose. At the word "go," they have to race to be the first to put on their stocking (over their pants).
❑ This alternative allows the socks to be reused after playing. Ask each guest to bring a pair of inexpensive baby socks to the shower. Then separate each pair and toss them all into a pile. Players race to be the first to find three matching pairs. Or, give players 10 seconds to find as many pairs as they can.

Take airing the laundry to task.

When
before/after baby is born

How
String a five foot (or longer) clothesline across a room if playing indoors, or across two posts if playing outside. You'll also need a cordless phone, a baby doll, a laundry basket of baby clothing, and a bag of wooden clothespins.

Set the bag of clothespins in the laundry basket and place the laundry basket by the clothesline. Call up a clotheshorse to play, the domestic diva has one minute to hold the cordless phone under their ear, burp baby, and hang as much clothing on the clothesline as they can. If the multi-tasker drops the baby or phone or time runs out, their turn ends.

Count each item of clothing hung as you remove them and return the clothing back to the basket. Select two additional chore masters to take their turns at this garment grind. The most prolific clothes hanger of the three wins.

Variation/Tips
- Depending on your budget, fill the basket with baby clothes salvaged from a thrift shop, a new bag of baby socks and washcloths, or new complete duds (to give to mom after).
- If you have a small gathering, ask each attendee to go a round on the clothesline.
- Make the game more difficult by blindfolding each plainclothes player before they start.

DIDN'T MEAN TO BURST YOUR BUBBLE

Ankle-biters rule in this popping game.

When
before/after baby is born

How
Tie one fully inflated balloon to everybody's right ankle. At the word go, everybody tries to burst everyone else's bubble by stomping on it and at the same time protect their own bubble. If your balloon gets popped, you are out of the game. Last bubble buster standing with their balloon intact wins.

Variation/Tips
❏ Try to outline the boundaries for this game so any balloonaticks can't cheat by simply running away from the action. You can arrange chairs to form a square that players with un-popped balloons have to stay within.

❏ Give two players one helium balloon each that's tethered to an equal length of ribbon. They have to tie the balloon to one wrist. Give each player a butterfly net. They have three minutes to try to net the other player's butterfly (the balloon).

DOCTOR'S ORDERS

A frantic prescription to follow directions.

When
before/after baby is born

How
Before the party, write a fictional short story about mom's pregnancy that is filled with occurrences of the words "RIGHT" and "LEFT." For example: She would have LEFT for the doctor's earlier, but she LEFT her keys by the door and had to turn RIGHT around. Then she remembered the RIGHT key was actually RIGHT in the car seat next to her....

Pick someone who won't be playing, like mom or host, to read the story aloud. Guests stand in a circle, randomly give a diaper to two people in the circle. Whenever a diaper holder hears RIGHT, that person gives the diaper to the individual on their right. If the diaper holder hears LEFT, player gives the diaper to the person on their left, and so on. There are always two people holding a diaper until instructed to pass it right or left. The person left holding the bag—er, diaper holds the right prescription for victory.

Variation/Tips
- If you don't have a way with words, just make up a story and randomly insert the words RIGHT or LEFT throughout. Be very generous with the insertions, you'll want to have several instances of one direction and different combinations. For example: Never feed LEFT, LEFT, RIGHT peanut butter to a LEFT, RIGHT, RIGHT, LEFT baby.
- Instead of passing only when a direction is indicated, have players pass at constant intervals, changing direction only when instructed by the story.
- For this variation, give everybody a clean diaper, but include one that is secretly marked inside (with a little chocolate syrup)

before playing. Everybody passes their diaper in the direction dictated by the story at the same time. At the end of the story, the group opens their diapers, whoever has the dirty one is the winner.

❑ Another variation that plays with one diaper: create a list of instructions and tape to a wrapped gift. Each person who gets the diaper then reads off the next line. For example, "Give to the person who was last to arrive." and pass the gift to that person. Continue with at least 10 more instructions like "Give to the nearest person with black hair, Give to the youngest person, etc." until the last line instructs the winning player to keep the gift. See the Onion Peeling Variation in the Appendix for a set of rhyming instructions.

❑ Or, pass on the passing entirely and give out a score sheet to guests that instructs them to add or subtract points based on what's applicable. For example, "Are you wearing pantyhose? Add 10 points. Were you the last to arrive? Subtract 25 points. Count the number of buttons you have, add 5 points for each button. Were you a boy/girl scout? Add 10 points. If you can shout out 'She's having a baby!' Add 10 points. Have waist-length hair? Add 15 points. Wearing pearls? Add 15 points. Are you wearing running shoes? Subtract 10 points." And so on. (You could include esoteric facts that only apply to specific individuals for great conversation later.) Whoever has the most points in the end wins the game.

❑ This version of pass the item "penalizes" instead of rewards the player caught with the item. Put a plastic shower cap inside a small paper bag (tape closed) for passing. Tell players that whoever ends up with the bag has to model what's inside for the group—don't tell them what it is, just hint that it's a flimsy item perfect for the shower. Suddenly that bag gets passed around very quickly!

DON'T WAKE THE BABY

Quietly tiptoe your way to victory.

When
before/after baby is born

How
You'll need two baby rattles and two contestants. Tie one rattle to each player's knee. The rattle rivals go to one end of the room. The goal is to be the first to reach the other side of the room and touch the wall without making any noise.

The rest of the movers and shakers watch to make sure not a peep is made during the dash. If a player's rattle makes noise, send the loud mouth back to start over. Award a silent victory to your quiet as a mouse winner.

Variation/Tips
- Players are not allowed to touch their rattle with their hands during the race.
- Organize additional rounds for more people who want to shake, rattle, and roll (or rather, avoid doing so).
- Shake things up by adding a second rattle to the player's ankle.
- If baby rattles aren't on hand, try jingle bells.
- A variation of this game is to have five alarm clocks hidden in the house to go off at the same time. Give players one minute to find and mute all the alarms.

IN PLAIN SIGHT

Practice seeing what's right in front of you.

When
before/after baby is born

How
Send the party out of the room for a minute. Place a baby thermometer in plain but not completely obvious sight (on the edge of a table or on the floor at the base of a TV, for example).

Call them back in. They have to find the baby thermometer in the room. First one to retrieve the thermometer wins the right to hide it for the next round. Repeat as enthusiasm allows.

Variation/Tips
❑ Remind searchers that the thermometer is in plain sight, they do not have to open drawers or cabinets to search for it.
❑ If players are having a hard time seeing the forest for the trees, declare a one minute warning before ending the game. Show everyone where the thermometer was and start anew.
❑ Don't have a baby thermometer? Use a sewing thimble instead.
❑ Another way to play: stand everybody in a circle, pick one person to be the Guesser. Give a thimble to one player in the circle, this player passes it to another player with one hand behind their back while pretending to pass it to another with the other hand. Everybody in the circle of life is pretending or actually passing the thimble around. After 40 seconds, stop. The Guesser has to point to the person who has the thimble.

IT'S A WRAP

Changing diapers becomes a lesson in side by side parenting.

When
before/after baby is born

How
You'll need two baby dolls (or stuffed animals), two cloth diapers, two bottles of baby powder, and a handful of safety pins to play. Assemble the materials on a table or countertop.

Select four players to partner up and form two teams. The two teams race to be the fastest to diaper their baby to win. The only rule is that each pair has to do this while standing side by side and holding hands. This leaves one person with a free left hand and their teammate with a free right hand. The wrapping partners work together with their free hands to powder and diaper their baby.

Variation/Tips
- To avoid a big mess, instruct teams to pantomime the sprinkling of baby powder (tape the opening closed just in case).
- For more of a challenge, pre-diaper each baby. Teams have to remove the old diaper before they can put on a new one.
- A simpler variation: instead of diapering the dolls, teams race to put on the baby's socks and shoes.
- In lieu of making a pair hold hands, have them place one hand behind their back.
- Or, have one-on-one diaper dashes, but each player can only use one hand to diaper or must diaper while blindfolded.
- Individuals may use both hands, but use cloth diapers and safety pins to diaper a balloon without popping the balloon.
- Instead of diapering the dolls, have players race to swaddle their baby correctly. See Appendix for swaddling instructions.
- Forget about diapering, have pairs race to be first to put on each other's shoes and successfully tie the laces!

MOBILE MOMMIES

Speed strolling with baby.

When
before/after baby is born

How
To conduct this outdoor baby stroller chase, you'll need a cheap baby stroller and a baby doll (a toy store will have both). Create a short obstacle course with furniture or cones that strollers must roll their way through. You could also place a broomstick across the path at chest level to force players to duck under the obstacle.

Your stroller rollers take turns racing the path with a baby in their carriage. Time how long it takes each pushy parent to finish. A speed stroller is disqualified if baby falls out of their stroller during the run. Quickest legwork wins.

Variation/Tips
❑ In lieu of an obstacle course, use chalk to draw a crooked route on the ground that players have to follow. The route should take at least 20 steps to walk and have many twists and turns.

❑ Make this a moonlight move. Give your stroller a sheet of newspaper rolled into a large cone. The player holds the cone up like a megaphone, but backwards, and puts her head in the large opening so that she is looking out the cone's small opening (make it about 2 inches in diameter). Time each cone-head's attempt to finish the same route.

Scramble to spoon a little yolk.

When
before/after baby is born

How
You'll need six raw eggs and teaspoons to play. Select six baby sitters to line up. Give each sitter one egg and spoon, they must cradle their baby with the spoon only. Encourage your egg minders to name their little yolk. The goal is to be the first to whisk their baby 12 feet (about two body lengths) to the crib (an empty egg carton on a table). No touching the baby with anything but a spoon. Baby is considered tucked into bed when the egg is deposited safely into an open spot in the egg carton. Get set, scramble!

Any sitters who crack up by doing the Humpty Dumpty (go splat with their eggs) are eliminated from the game. Encourage observers to cheer on their favorite baby wrangler.

Variation/Tips

❑ This should be played outdoors. You can use hard-boiled eggs to make accidents less messy and more palatable for indoor play, but part of the fun is risking messy matters.

❑ Fill some of the spaces in the empty carton with eggs so that not everyone who makes it to the crib can actually fit in.

❑ Stand players in a tight circle, they autograph one of three hard boiled eggs to make it "their" baby. They toss the eggs back and forth in the circle. After every third throw, everyone takes one step backward. Game ends when an egg hits the ground.

❑ A sit-down variation: sit eggheads at a small table, but blindfold them. Put each of their eggs in a small cup. They transfer their egg from their cup to an empty spot in an egg carton at the center of the table. They may use their hands to feel their way to the crib.

QUADRUPLETS

Caring for multiple stork deliveries.

When
before/after baby is born

How
To prepare, you'll need eight dolls (or stuffed animals) and baby props like diapers, baby powder, a milk bottle, a baby outfit, etc. Pin a nametag with unique name on each baby. Create a to-do task, one for each baby, such as John needs his diaper changed, Mary needs to be fed her milk bottle, Mark needs a change of clothes and so on.

Pick someone from the group to go up against Mom. Each player gets four babies and they have to share the baby goods between them. Inform the players that they will race to see who can take care of their babies the fastest. Read the task list out loud to the caretakers and at the word "go," they have to recall their tasks and act fast. Person who completes the most tasks correctly wins.

Variation/Tips
❑ To prevent cheating, arrange the players so that they're facing away from each other (or back to back) and can't see what's being done to the other babies.
❑ If the budget allows, double the number of dolls and make up additional tasks to double the fun.
❑ Have observers write how long they think it'll take each mom to accomplish her tasks (pass around a sheet of paper, have them write their name next to their guess).
❑ A nice follow-up on this game is to quiz players on multiple births. What do you call 2 babies born at once? Twins. The rest are: 3 (triplets), 4 (quadruplets), 5 (quintuplets), 6 (sextuplets), 7 (septuplets), 8 (octuplets), 9 (nonuplets), 10 (decaplets), 11 (undecaplets), and 12 (dodecaplets).

Players wait on pins and needles to play this game.

When
before/after baby is born

How
You'll need a baby bottle and a bunch of large safety pins. Players take turns standing over the open baby bottle and dropping as many safety pins as they can into the bottle. As soon as they miss a pin, their turn ends and the next competitor takes their shot. Record the number of pins successfully dropped by each pinhead. Pin the win on whoever bottles the most pins.

Variation/Tips
- ❏ Weigh down the bottle or have someone hold it in place to prevent tipping.
- ❏ Limit it so that players have to hold the pin at waist level or higher before dropping the pin.
- ❏ If players are having a difficult time getting pins into the bottle, allow each player a one minute time limit to drop as many pins into the bottle as they can.
- ❏ Run a tiebreaker round if needed.
- ❏ Give the bottle and pins to mom afterward.
- ❏ Try using wooden clothespins instead of safety pins.
- ❏ A harder game: have players start three feet from the baby bottle. While holding a wooden clothespin between their legs, they waddle up to the bottle and then drop the pin into the bottle. You may need to weigh down the bottle with some sand to prevent it from tipping. Because this is so difficult, not many players will score. Give each player three tries.

ROCK THE BABY

Try to be the last one passing off this hot potato.

When
before/after baby is born

How
You'll need two baby dolls, a portable tape or CD player, and an audio tape or CD of baby lullabies. The host or a volunteer will need to sit out to run the game.

Players stand in a circle. Give one baby doll to a player in the circle and the other baby doll to a player on the opposite side of the circle. Guests pass the baby (each goes in the opposite direction) as music plays (try to differentiate the babies with some different colored ribbon so it's always clear which baby goes in what direction). Stop the music at random times. Whoever is caught holding a baby takes a time-out from the group. Play continues. When you're down to two players, take out one of the babies. The last one to pass the babe off before the music ends wins.

Variation/Tips
❑ If your guests are especially nimble, require guests to pass babies using their knees only, no hands allowed!
❑ Mom can be the one controlling the music. Or, if she'd rather join in on the fun, recruit a volunteer to play the music while mom plays.
❑ Instead of dolls, try teddy bears.
❑ Turn to Minding Your Fruits & Vegetables and Doctor's Orders for more variations on the "pass the present" type game.

RUSH DELIVERY

Practicing the dash to the hospital.

When
before/after baby is born

How
Create a start line and finish line about 10 feet (or the length of one and a half persons) away. Blow up two round 10" balloons. Divide contestants into two teams, then form each into a column at the starting point. Give the heads of each team an inflated balloon to hold between their thighs.

The object of the game is to get to the hospital (the finish line) first without dropping their baby (the balloon) before they reach the hospital. Once they reach the hospital, they must labor to deliver the baby (drop the balloon) without using their hands. This can get quite tricky because the balloon acquires static cling during the trip. The relay repeats with the next member of their team until all members have had a run or a five minute time limit runs out. Bragging rights go to the team with the most successful trips.

Variation/Tips
❏ In lieu of team competitions, have a pair of players compete at a time.
❏ Put a laundry basket at the end of each finish line. Players drop the baby (without using their hands) into the "crib."
❏ If players are really adventurous and dressed for it, give them water balloons to deliver to the hospital. If they break their water on the way, they're eliminated from the game.
❏ An easier game has two players racing to deliver potatoes instead of balloons between their thighs (anywhere above the knee). Player who delivers the most babies on one run to the hospital the fastest wins. You'll need about 30 raw baking potatoes for two players to play at a time.

SAFE TO EAT

Sitters clap for baby safe foods.

When
before/after baby is born

How
Players stand in a line and choose one to be the Baby. Baby faces the line and shouts out a variety of things that he or she wants to eat. The group indicates if it's edible by clapping twice in front of their chest. If it's not for eating, they clap once behind their back. They always clap an answer immediately following every item named.

Baby starts by listing random things about a second apart, like this: "blanket... ball... banana..." After each word, players clap their answer. If a player answers incorrectly (for example, claps edible when the item is inedible) or takes too long to clap, that player is eliminated. Baby should gradually speak faster to make the game harder, "apple, chicken, money, honey, candy, bunny, brick—broom—baseball— blueberries..." pausing to eliminate players who are caught tripping up along the way. The last player left gets to eat up their victory.

Variation/Tips
- If it's too difficult to clap behind your back, have players clap above their heads for "edible," and by the knees for "not edible."
- Make it easier to hear incorrect answers, have players clap once for edible and snap their fingers once for inedible.
- The Baby can create a list beforehand and read off the list of items. Add a spotter to help catch players making mistakes.
- Some foods are not appropriate for feeding to babies, such as honey or peanut butter. In these situations, the correct answer is "not edible."
- If the game goes for a while without any mistakes, suggest a lightning round or declare the remaining players winners.

SNIFFLES

A test for tissue excavation engineers.

When
before/after baby is born

How
You'll need three square shaped boxes of tissues for this game. Select three people to play. Say that mom has caught the sniffles and will need a whole lot of tissues. The player's job is to remove all the tissues from the tissue box (one at a time) as quickly as they can.

Whoever empties their box first wins.

Variation/Tips
- This quiet game is a nice distraction for those not enthusiastic about watching mom open presents.
- If multiple tissues are accidentally pulled out at once during the race, the player has to separate the clumped tissues before resuming removing more tissues from the box.
- Once all the tissue boxes have been emptied, have the same contestants race to see who can be the first to successfully cram all their tissues back into the box.

SPILT MILK

There's no crying over spilt milk in this race.

When
before/after baby is born

How
You'll need two small baby jars that have been emptied and cleaned, and two coffee mugs filled with milk. Set up this game outdoors by placing two small tables 10 feet apart. Put the two milk mugs and two teaspoons on one table and two empty baby jars on the other table.

Select two milkmaids to play. Their job is spoon milk from the coffee mug, run the distance between the two tables, and pour whatever's still in their spoon into the baby jar. Whoever fills their baby jar to overflowing first with milk has milked their way to a win.

Variation/Tips
❑ Reset the game for additional rounds if more milkmaids want to play.
❑ If you're pressed for space, play this indoor alternative. Seat players on a kitchen counter, players have to transfer milk from the mug to the jar (set one foot apart) on the counter in front of them using a spoon or eye dropper.
❑ Yet another variation, fill small tea cups (get the kid-sized plastic ones for playtime if you can) to the brim with milk. Have players race 15 feet (about the length of two-and-a-half persons) to a finish line while holding the cup. First person across the line with the most milk remaining in their cup wins. You may want to use a food scale to determine the winner.
❑ If you don't want to use fresh milk, create a milk lookalike with a couple tablespoons of cornstarch and a cup of water. Or, you can substitute sugar for the milk.

SPOONING THE PUDDING

Proof of the pudding is definitely in the eating.

When
before/after baby is born

How
Call up four players and pair them into two teams. Give one member of each team an individual serving sized pudding cup and a plastic spoon. At the word "Go!" the two teams race to feed pudding to their partner, the team that finishes their pudding first wins. Simple, right? Just one thing, the feeder on each team has to wear a blindfold before the feeding frenzy begins.

Variation/Tips
❑ Give players bibs made of plastic trash bags to keep their clothing clean (cut a hole in the bottom of the bag that's big enough for a head to fit through, pull the bag over your body). You'll want to play this outside or line the floor under the players with newspaper for easy clean-up.

❑ To make this pudding pursuit even more difficult, blindfold both the feeder and the eater. Recruit two judges to watch each team and call out when they've finished spooning their pudding.

TYING THE CORD

A race to collect the most umbilical cords.

When
before/after baby is born

How
Before the party prep: cut lots of different lengths of pink and blue yarn (at least five times the number of invited guests). Scatter the cut yarn pieces in plain sight throughout the house.

To play, have guests pair up into teams to collect as many pieces of yarn (doesn't matter which color) as they can and tie them together all within a five minute period. Whichever team has the longest length of yarn in the end is the winner.

Variation/Tips
❑ After the winner is declared, tell players to see whether they have more blue or pink yarn, that's the sex of their "baby."
❑ If you're not comfortable having guests roam the whole house, confine the game to one room and place yarn in that room only.
❑ Save this game for last, letting guests stumble upon the yarn in the course of the party. Do not explain what the yarn is for until you're ready to play—some will collect them, others will just ignore them. Then surprise them all by revealing how the game is played.
❑ This variation is a simple scavenger game. You'll need a bunch (twice the number of guests is ideal) of tiny baby rattles or plastic babies (usually available at the baby shower or cake decorating section of craft stores) or baby socks. Hide them in various places in one room. Give guests five minutes to find the item, whoever locates and collects the most wins.

WEE GULPS

Nursing a drink to success.

When
before/after baby is born

How
You'll need three sippy cups, apple juice, and three pairs of players. Fill all the cups halfway with juice. One player on each team has to feed the juice to their partner; the partner's job is to drink as quickly as possible without using their hands. The team to gulp down their sippy cup first wins.

Variation/Tips
☐ Some people like to use baby bottles with the nipples instead of a cup for the full experience.

☐ Substitute soda or milk for juice.

☐ To play a prank on one of your players, place some plastic wrap over the opening of the bottle before screwing on the nipple. When the player with the prank bottle tries to drink it, nothing will come out no matter how hard they suckle.

☐ A creative way to draft players is to play a hot potato type game. Gather everybody around and distribute three cups to hold. Play some baby music and have them pass the cups around. Whoever is stuck with a cup when you stop the music is selected to play—and gets to select a partner.

ZOO KEEPER

Some monkey business in cookie sorting.

When
before/after baby is born

How
This game is easiest to play while sitting down at a table. Give each player a box (individual serving size) of animal cookies. At the word "go," players go ape by opening their box and sorting their menagerie of animals by species (all bears, all giraffes, etc.). Fastest sorter in this rat race wins. Heap the lion's share of praise on your winner.

Variation/Tips
❑ If you don't want to buy every guest a box of animal cookies, buy just three and select three individuals to play. A cost-effective alternative is to buy animal cookies in bulk and then dole out two cups worth of cookies to each player.

❑ After declaring your fastest sorter, bestow a prize on whoever has the most of each different species (incomplete parts of a cookie don't count). Award multiple prizes if there's a tie.

❑ To get more mileage out of each box of animal cookies, have players stand five feet from their empty box and see who can toss the most number of cookies back into their box.

❑ Another way to play with these treats, set aside one of each kind of animal (it should be a whole, unbroken cookie) and place inside a paper bag. Have three players take turns reaching into the bag and retrieving an animal (the group decides what kind) by touch only. For example, if the group agrees to ask for a gorilla, player has to catch a gorilla to earn a point. Go in rounds to see who has the lightest (and most accurate) touch. (And yes, discard the cookies afterward.)

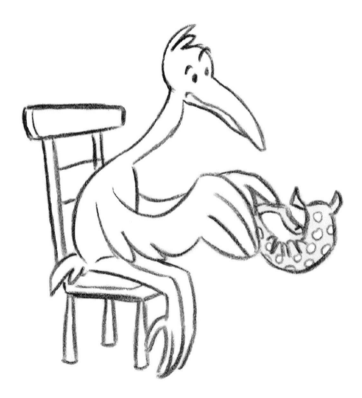

SIT DOWN GAMES

BABES IN TOYLAND

Toying with child's play.

When
before/after baby is born

How
Toy around a toy store catalog before the shower. Cut out ten pictures total of children's playthings, well-known and less-known ones. Tape the pictures to individual pieces of paper and number each item. Keep an answer key of names to each toy.

To play, players guess the name of each toy by writing down their answers on a piece of paper. Read off your answer key for playmates to check their answers. Whoever correctly identifies the most toys wins.

Variation/Tips
❑ To make the game easier, type up a list of toy names (including some that aren't in the group of pictures) and provide this to guests so they can match a name to each toy.

BEDTIME STORY

Paging through story time.

When
before/after baby is born

How
This is a very easy, quiet game that anybody can play! You'll need a thick book of children's bedtime stories and a bookmark for this game. Let the group have a good look at the book and tell them how many pages are in the book.

Randomly insert a bookmark into the book. Players have to guess what page the bookmark is now in. Your bookworms may look at the closed book, but they cannot open it. Whoever comes closest to the page with the bookmark has booked victory.

Variation/Tips
❑   If you want to offer more opportunities to award winners, pair players up. Insert the bookmark in a different place for each pair, then each player has a 50-50 chance of winning. For this variation, you may want to stipulate that their guess has to be the closest without going past the page.

❑   If you don't have a children's book handy, you can always substitute a dictionary. And fashion a bookmark out of a folded piece of paper.

Mom's turn to reach out and touch someone.

When
before/after baby is born

How
Ask all guests to come wearing a maternity dress (or oversized shirt) with a pillow stuffed underneath. When it's time to open presents, have everyone replace their pillow with the gift they brought. Mom of the hour is now a doctor, she has to feel each guest's tummy and guess what the present is.

Variation/Tips
- After everyone's arrived, take a group picture for laughs.
- To make the game more competitive and interesting to your players, try this variation: every time mom makes an incorrect guess, award a small chocolate or other token prize to the gift giver (who then reveals the present).
- Remind guests a day or two before the party that they'll be playing this game. Encourage them to wrap gifts without their packaging to create more odd shapes.
- Or, supply small baby items to free guests of having to bring anything. Have guests tuck their item on top of their pillow under their shirts for mom to feel and identify.

BOTTOMS UP

Score points by getting derrieres in the air.

When
before/after baby is born

How
You'll need eight plastic babies from the craft or cake decorating supply store. You only want the babies that are sitting up.

Put the babies in a large plastic cup. Players take turns shaking the cup and pouring out the babies onto a table (like dice). The object is to get two or more that land stomach down so that the babies are in a "bottoms up" position. Depending on how big the group of players is, you may want to let them go three to five rounds, writing down how many "bottoms up" a player gets with each roll. The bottom line: highest score at the end of all the rounds is tops.

Variation/Tips
❏ Give a bonus of 10 points if any babies end up stacked on top of each other.
❏ This variation only requires a pair of dice, a sippy cup, and several wrapped prizes (the number of gifts depends on your budget, but it should be less than the number of guests). Sit players in a circle with gifts piled in the center. Use a timer to count down 10 minutes. During this time, players take turns rolling the dice after shaking it in a sippy cup. Anybody who rolls doubles may select a gift. If no doubles are rolled, player loses chance at a gift. In either scenario, the cup and dice must be passed to the next player to try.

If all the gifts are claimed before time is up, the next player to roll doubles may steal a gift from another player. At the end of the 10 minutes, whoever is still holding a gift (or two) wins that gift and keeps it.

Game that rewards the nesting instinct.

When
before/after baby is born

How
Before the party, use crayons to decorate each egg with a baby face. You'll need enough eggs so that there is one for each attendee.

Pile the eggs in a bowl by the entrance. As guests arrive, tell each arrival to take a little yolk under their wing by selecting an egg. They should sign their adopted egg with a pen so we know who is the nanny of each egg. Your nannies are to chaperone their chick for the duration of the party and tend the egghead as they deem fit.

Don't mention the babies again until the end of the party. Before guests take their leave, reveal the purpose of this game: whoever still has their egg (unbroken and not forgotten) wins a small prize.

Variation/Tips
- Hard boil the eggs beforehand to reduce the risk of a messy accident, or substitute plastic eggs.
- If guests ask what to do with their babies during the course of the shower, reply that it's their baby to chaperone as they please.
- If you have the time and inclination, decorate the eggs more elaborately, giving each unique characteristics. Guests are more inclined to keep the egghead as a party favor.
- If you come across unattended babies, collect them in a secret "nursery" until the end of the game. Give the parents of these latchkey eggs some friendly ribbing.

CHILDPROOF

Identify the household dangers lurking inside this bad egg.

When
before/after baby is born

How
You'll need a large plastic, opaque egg (like the ones used to sell panty hose). Before the party, go around the home to collect small objects you wouldn't want a baby to pick up (a pin, paperclip, nail, staple, gum, marble, etc.) and place in the egg. Try to pick at least 10 different objects that will fit in the egg, the more the better.

When you're ready to play, give guests pen and paper. Pass the egg around, telling them that inside the egg—which they're not allowed to open—are dangerous things collected from around the house that should be kept away from a baby. Their job is to guess what those items are inside the egg. Give them 5 minutes to get their egg on.

When time's up, open the goose egg and reveal its contents. Whoever has the most matching items on their list wins.

Variation/Tips
❑ If the plastic egg doesn't seal tightly, tape it closed to prevent the egg from popping open while it's being handled. Cut to open.
❑ Guests may rattle the egg in hopes of identifying items by sound. Make sure the egg is passed all around so that everybody gets their fair shake.
❑ Another way to play, get half a dozen plastic Easter eggs and place only one baby-hazardous item (such as a pin) or baby safety item (such as an outlet cover) in each egg. Players pass around the eggs and try to determine what's inside each egg without opening it.

LIVING

bringing up baby.

en
baby is born

w
:sities, like diapers, baby wipes,
le, etc. Save the receipt, you'll
ce tags from the items before
ith a blanket.

love the blanket from the baby
to calculate the total cost for all
nan has his price figured out, let
:on whose price is right (closest
' over) cashes in on the win.

/Tips
iduals guess the price of each
the correct price earns a point.
the tie gets a point. The one

adruplets and Baby Sitting
be reused.
baby things, guess the cost of
0 colleges (a mix of public and
'om your list one at a time,
the annual tuition for each
n amounts and give the player
oint. Most points wins. You can
ound your area or make it mom's
. (Use the internet to look up
I colleges before playing.)

COUNT OFF

Play the numbers with a baby food jar.

When
before/after baby is born

How
You'll need a clean baby food jar and a bunch of large safety pins. Fill the jar with safety pins, counting the exact number you put in. Write the number inside the baby food jar lid, write small so that it's not easily visible, and screw the lid closed over the jar.

Ask guests to write their name and the number of pins they think are in the jar on an index card. Keep a little shoebox (or big envelope) by the jar so that anyone who's down for the count can leave their guesswork in the box.

When all your calculating minds have had a chance to crunch the numbers, open the jar and read the number inside the jar lid. The written guess that comes closest to the actual count wins.

Variation/Tips
❑ Instead of safety pins, substitute mini jelly beans, mini candy pacifiers, mom's favorite candy, or cotton balls or swabs, or whatever your imagination desires.
❑ Fill several jars with different items in each, and let people take a shot at predicting the count of each jar.
❑ Or, have players estimate how many slices are in one jar of sliced pickles. Count it in front of everyone after votes are cast.
❑ Fill a jar with coins and folded up money in various denominations. Attendees try to deduce the total dollar amount inside.
❑ Try filling a pair of baby shoes or a small baby feeding bottle.
❑ To help you easily address thank you notes after the party, ask guests to also write down their address on the index card.

CRIB SHEETS

Identify players by their growing pains.

When
before/after baby is born

How
Pass out a pen and sheet of lined paper to each guest. At the top of the page, everybody writes three facts about their babyhood, such as when they started talking, how much they weighed at birth, maybe they were a C-section baby, had colic, or refused a pacifier, etc. Ask players not to share or discuss this information during the game.

When all the facts are down, players draw a big T under their facts, and write "Guess" on the left side of the T and "Guesser" on the right side of the T. Collect the crib sheets, post them on a wall.

Everybody goes to each page to read over the baby facts and write the name of the person they think that baby grew up to be (under Guess) and print their own name (on the Guesser side).

The game emcee goes to one page and reads off the three facts. The player being described should identify him/herself. Emcee puts a check mark beside the name of each correct Guesser. Continue with the rest of the pages. Tally up the scores, declare the player with the most correct answers the winner.

Variation/Tips
❑ Remind crib mates to write their name on the same line as their guess.
❑ This game is ideal for a well acquainted, smaller group of guests.
❑ If all your guests have birthed at least one child, have every parent write two unique facts about their baby's delivery instead. For example, no epidural was used, the baby was a breech birth; or labor lasted 20 hours, baby was born at home, etc.

CRY BABIES

Contestants cry like a baby then play it by ear.

When
before/after baby is born

How
You'll need a tape recorder and a blank tape to set-up the game. Early in the gathering, randomly select 6 to 8 guests one at a time to go into another room (away from the party) to record their imitation of a baby. Assign each recording a number (record the number, then record the cry). Keep a master list to identify your cry babies.

After you've recorded enough baby bellows, give a piece of paper and pen to all your invitees (including those who recorded a cry). Play each recording, pausing for audio auditors to write who they think the good cry belongs to. After you've played all the recordings, replay the tape while identifying each baby boomer. Get the most correct answers to demonstrate good sound judgment.

Variation/Tips
❏ Wait about 15 minutes after making the last recording to give any sharp-eyed guests a chance to forget the order in which you made the tape recording.
❏ If this is taking place after the baby is already born, try to get a recording of the baby's actual cry before the shower starts and let that be recording number one to throw off guests.
❏ This variation is much simpler, but requires guests to be more outgoing. Guests take turns imitating a baby cry one at a time in front of the group. Invitees clap for the best cry. The one who most sounds like a babe by group consensus gets to cry out in joy.

DIAPER DUTY

Decipher dirty diapers to get the poop.

When
before/after baby is born

How
Before the party set-up: buy seven to ten different candy bars and cut in half (save or discard the other half). Place the half bar on a clean microwave plate and microwave it 30 seconds or until it just starts to melt. Spoon the soft candy onto the inside of a clean diaper, repeat with the others, putting a different candy bar in each diaper. Make sure you number or color-code the diapers and keep a master answer key.

To play, line up the open diapers on a table. Challenge everyone to identify the candy bar in each open diaper. Let the group work together to deduce each diaper's contents. It's up to you to decide if you want to allow tasting.

Variation/Tips
❑ For a more individualized competition, pass out pen and paper for players to write their answers. Once everybody's hazarded a guess, read the answer key aloud so players can score themselves.
❑ Instead of melting the candy bar, use your hands to mash each full bar into a tight ball and center each ball in a diaper.
❑ As an alternative to candy, spoon a couple tablespoons of different baby foods into each diaper and have participants identify each baby food.
❑ Or, test your player's sense of smell instead. Mash or smear a different food (banana, chocolate, mustard, tomato sauce, cheese, tuna, coffee, peanut butter, onions, vanilla) in each diaper and seal the openings (try stapling the edge). Ask guests to sniff out the scent emanating from each diaper.

HOUSEHOLD GOODS

Judging a product by its cover.

When
before/after baby is born

How
To prepare for this game of fighting dirty, gather six to eight brand name cleaning products from around the house (or purchase some for variety), such as dishwashing soap, floor cleaner, window cleaner, toilet cleaner, dust remover, etc. Remove the labels or cover it with a black piece of construction paper. Write a unique number on each product. Assemble on a tray or table.

Give players a pen and piece of paper. The goal is to identify the name of each product by its container. Whoever sweeps in the most correct answers comes clean with a win!

Variation/Tips
❏ If desired, take your guests to the cleaners by giving them a list of all the brand names represented by the containers (and maybe a few that aren't) to select from.
❏ Remove the paper to reveal the labels on each product. Group players into teams of two or three people, each team has five minutes to write a story that incorporates as many of the products as possible. See Minding Your Fruits & Vegetables, instead of writing a veggie tale, write a clean story. Mom picks her favorite.

LIL' MUGS

See who has the sharpest eye for babes.

When
before/after baby is born

How
Tell invitees to bring a color copy of a picture of themselves as a baby—the younger the better. Collect the pictures as guests arrive.

Use children's alphabet magnets to affix each picture with a unique letter of the alphabet to the refrigerator door. Distribute a copy of the guest list and pen to your players. Their job is to match the attendees to the babies on the fridge door (by writing the letter next to the name of the person they think the baby is). To announce the answers, point to each baby photo one at a time and have the grown up step forward to collect their picture. Player with the most correct matches gets to mug for the camera.

Variation/Tips
❑ Ask invitees to mail (or email) a color copy of their baby photo, that way you'll have them all before the party and nobody worries about losing a valuable picture.

❑ If a party pooper "forgets" to submit a baby photo, have them draw a picture of themselves as a baby and use for the game.

❑ If invitees don't know each other very well or you have a large gathering, ask people to provide a recent picture of themselves too. Post the recent pictures up on one half of the fridge door and the baby pictures on the other half of the door.

❑ If you're really craft-handy, cut out silhouettes of a pregnant mother and place the baby photo inside the belly of each cut-out. Proceed with play as usual.

❑ This twist is for a star-struck crowd: research the internet or gossip magazines for baby pictures of famous celebrities. Test your star gazers' ability to identify the famous baby mugs.

MOM'S PRIDE & JOY

Measuring up mom.

When
before baby is born

How
This game is most fun with a mom-to-be who's at ease with her womanly curves during her pregnancy. Pass out a spool of ribbon and scissors to your guests. They're to cut the length of material they think will go around the circumference of mom's tummy.

After everybody's taken some ribbon, mom wraps a piece of ribbon (of a different color) around her tummy and cuts the correct length. Pass this around for guests to see how their ribbon measures up. Whoever comes closest wins.

Variation/Tips
❑ If mom is feeling sensitive about her body, she might like some of the variations on the next page.
❑ You can substitute toilet paper or string. Some people also like to use yarn, but it's not very accurate because the material can be stretched.
❑ Another way to play: pre-cut different lengths of ribbon (including one that matches mom's circumference) and number each one and tape to a wall. Have guests pick the ribbon they think fits around mom.
❑ Or, use a spool of uncut ribbon and have guests sign their name anywhere along the length of the ribbon that matches the length of mom's circumference. Then have mom try on the ribbon.
❑ You can lengthen game play by having players also take lengths of material that they think will constitute the circumference of mom's thigh and wrist.
❑ If you don't want to use string or ribbon, just ask guests to write down their best guess on mom's tummy circumference on individual pieces of paper.

- This variation is perfect for after the baby's arrived—players guess the baby's total length, length of the baby finger, waist circumference, and length of a foot.
- A playful twist on this game starts with passing out a roll of toilet paper to the group. Each person takes enough toilet paper that they believe is the equivalent to the circumference of daddy's waist. Players take turns bringing their toilet paper up to mom who then tries to wrap it around daddy's waist. Whoever's most accurate wins a prize.
- If dad is game, have players guess the circumference of daddy's flexed bicep, waist, thigh, his shoe size, height, etc.
- Extend the above variation further by having dad write down his specs, such as the circumference of his waist, on a scrap of paper, then insert it into a balloon. Blow up the balloon and place it underneath dad's shirt so it looks like he's expecting. After players write down what they think dad's circumference is. Dad delivers his baby and reveals the number to all. Whoever guessed the closest wins.
- Take the guesswork out of the game completely with this version. People take as much toilet paper as they would normally for the restroom. Each person then has to reveal one fact about themselves to the group for each square of paper they've taken. If the majority are shy of public speaking, ask gamers to pair up with someone they don't know well. Then give five minutes or so for all the pairs to proceed with the facts one-on-one.

MOMMY'S PURSE

A rummage through handbag haven.

When
before/after baby is born

How
Bring mommy's purse in front of the group. Do not open it. Players who want a shot at the prize purse have one minute to write down all the items they think are in mommy's money bag.

After the minute is up, mom loosens her purse strings and inventories the items she has in the bag before the group. The most accurate purse contents predictor is your winning bag lady.

Variation/Tips
❑ Warn mom before the party that this game will be played so she can discreetly remove private items from her purse.
❑ For a grab bag of fun: everyone sets their purse in front of them, then mom pulls out an item from hers. Your rummagers rush to be the first to produce a matching or similar item from their own purse. Mom continues pulling another seven or so items, one at a time. The bag handler who retrieves the most matching items first is the winner.
❑ A variation on the above variation: create then read off a list of items that purse owners have to race to produce from their own handbag first, such as something... pink/blue, that squeaks, sweet, crunchy, etc.

RANDOM WINNER

Practice random acts of kindness during the opening of presents.

When
before/after baby is born

How
This simple giveaway will entertain your present majority while mom is busy opening and appreciating her gifts.

Set a kitchen timer to go off every 5 minutes. Whoever's gift mom is opening when the timer rings is awarded a small prize. Assign a friend to diligently reset the timer each time it goes off and another to award prizes to the gifted winners.

Variation/Tips
❑ Tradition holds that the person who gave the seventh gift opened by mom will be the next to get pregnant. To take the pressure off of having mom pick the seventh gift to open, make note of the seventh guest to arrive and tag their gift. Then give the seventh gift to mom and make an announcement.

❑ A variation of this game is to play Gift Bingo. Give every guest a blank 5x5 grid bingo card before gift opening commences. Tell guests they are to fill in each square with a baby item they think mom will receive. The middle square is a free space. As mom opens her presents, players cross off any corresponding squares. When a player gets five across horizontally, vertically, or diagonally, they shout "bingo" and win a prize. The rest continue playing until there are no more presents.

❑ For a smaller shower, create a tic-tac-toe grid instead and play the same way as the bingo game above.

❑ A small prize can range from a gag gift (like a shower cap) to baby theme gift (a candy pacifier) to a tasty treat (a chocolate truffle) to the practical (dishwashing gloves). See the Appendix for more ideas.

SHOWER BAG

A baby game of touch and go.

When
before/after baby is born

How
You'll need to gather 10 items, one that begins with each letter of the words "Shower Bag." For example: Shades, Hat, Onesie, Washcloth, Egg, Ring, Bottle, Apple, Gloves. Put one item in each paper bag and write the letter it begins with on the bag. Assemble all the bags on the floor or table so that they spell out "Shower Bag."

Explain to guests they have to write what they think is in the paper bag. They may squeeze the bag but they cannot open it. The only hint they get is that the name of item begins with the letter written on its goodie bag. Whoever has the most accurate feelers bags the win.

Variation/Tips
❑ Alternatives to the suggested items: Sunscreen, Handbag, Orange, Wind-up toy, Elephant toy (stuffed animal), Rag, Brush, Alarm clock, Garment (as in an article of baby clothing).
❑ Or, do away with hints and simply number each bag.
❑ Instead of bags, put a different baby item in seven to ten disposable diapers (seal them up with tape to prevent peeking). Guests have to feel through the diaper to guess what they think is inside. Pick thicker diapers to make the game more challenging.
❑ A lengthier variation: write the alphabet on index cards, one letter per card. Then write a baby-related item that begins with each letter on the back of the corresponding card (A=applesauce, B=bib, C=crib, D=diapers, E=ear thermometer, F=feeding chair, G=gate, H=humidifier, I=iodine, J=jumpers, etc.). Players shout out items for each letter, whoever matches what's written gets to collect that calling card. Holder of the most trump cards wins this prediction game. If no one is able to guess the card up your sleeve, then no one collects that card.

STATS

Checking out the baby.

When
after baby is born

How
After everyone has had some time to see the baby, pass out a quiz that asks players to recall statistics about the newborn. You'll need copies of a game sheet prepared with these questions:

What is the baby's...?
weight
length
hair color
eye color
date of birth
time of birth
shirt color

Distribute the game sheet to attendees. Your baby visitors write their name across the top of their game sheet and fill in their estimates. Call on a couple offspring observers to volunteer their guess before revealing the correct answer to each question. Spotters earn a point for each correct answer (or closest to it). Whoever gets the most points earns the title of best baby watcher.

Variation/Tips
❑ Extend play further by asking baby observers to estimate any or all of the following baby measurements: circumference of head or wrist, how long the foot is, the length of a pinky finger, etc.
❑ If there are no clear winners, you may elect to award a prize to each player who got at least one answer correct.

STORK DELIVERY

Ordering up the ideal baby.

When
before baby is born

How
Recreate this game sheet for mom and each guest to fill out.

Guess which traits mom will choose for her stork delivery. Put an X under the appropriate column:

This baby will have...	Mom's	Dad's	
			hair
			eyes
			nose
			smile
			lips
			skin
			hands
			feet
			legs
			sense of humor
			patience
			brains
			creativity

When everyone's finished, have mom read off her selections. The person who has the most matches with mom wins.

Variation/Tips

❑ To personalize the game, add more personality/physical traits to the list that draw from mom and dad. Possibilities: sense of direction, style, cooking skills, organization, competitiveness, etc.

❑ Name an animal instead of mom/dad. For example, "This baby will have eyes like a ..." and "This baby will have the smarts of a ..."

SWEET TALK

Getting sweet on eye candy.

When
before/after baby is born

How
You'll need about eight different candies and paper plates. A real range of childhood favorites is ideal for playing this game. Besides candy bars, think butterscotch discs, licorice, chicken bones, and other hard candies from the past. Throw in some lesser known ones too such as the newer novelty candies that adults will be unfamiliar with. Disrobe the candy and put each on a separate paper plate, tape the wrapper under each corresponding plate to help you track the sweets. Write a unique number on each plate next to the treat.

To play, your sugar sleuths work together to determine the name of each naked confection by sight only. Once the group reaches consensus on a sweet nothing, reveal its identity. Repeat with the next plate until you've been through them all.

As a sweet reward for the sugar daddies and mommies, unleash them on the candy!

Variation/Tips
❏ Make this more competitive by having candy men and women individually write down their guesses on a piece of paper, then give points for each correct answer. Sweeten the pot with a prize for the player with the most correct answers.
❏ Hold a blind taste test. Cut each candy into bite-size cubes and have everybody taste it at the same time. The quickest to shout out the name of the treat wins that round.

WHO'S YOUR MOMMA

What do a foal, chick, and puppy call their momma?

When

before/after baby is born

How

This game tests how well players can match an adult animal to its infant form, for example: bear = cub, goose = gossling, cow = calf.

Create a game sheet with a list of animal babies on one column and then randomly list their adult form on another column. Make as many copies as you have guests. See Appendix for a sample game sheet and answer key. Pass out the game sheet, your momma matchers have one minute to draw lines matching the baby to its mummy. Read aloud the correct pairings so everyone can check their answers.

Variation/Tips

❑ Or, start with blank sheets of paper and pair players into teams. Paternity partners write down the names of as many animal babies as they know within two minutes. Most prolific team wins.

❑ Here's a variation to involve the guys: see who can list the most animal mascots from college sports. Then next to each mascot, list what that animal's baby would be.

❑ Or, chuck the pencil and paper and verbally quiz each player with the following "You're a <insert baby animal>, who's your momma?" See who's your most knowledgeable big momma.

❑ This variation requires a little more research to look up the answers beforehand. Guess the gestation period for each animal.

❑ Instead of quizzing for animal babies, query players on their creativity with baby things. For example: baby ocean : pond, baby plant : seed, baby rock : pebble, baby cookie : crumb, baby oat tree : acorn, etc.

WISDOM TEETH

Pull wisdom teeth for silly answers to parenting questions.

When
before/after baby is born

How
Cut a large wisdom tooth shape out of an index card. Make twice as many wisdom teeth as you have guests. Write a different question about raising children on each separate tooth, but write only as many questions as you have guests (you'll be left with an equal number of blank teeth). Some examples below (more in the Appendix):

- How do I make the smelly task of changing diapers less stinky?
- How do I find more time for sleep?
- What's a way to soothe a crying baby?
- How do I get a toddler to eat vegetables?
- How do parents decide who gets up for midnight feedings?

Give each person a blank tooth and a question tooth. Let players sink their teeth into the question by writing a brief answer to the parenting question they've received on the blank tooth. Collect the baby care questions in a paper bag and the answers in a separate bag.

Now the fun begins. Your tooth fairies take turns randomly extracting a question and answer card. All take a turn reading their wisdom teeth to the group. It might go something like this: "What's a way to soothe a crying baby? Flip a coin."

Variation/Tips
- For a more personal touch, have the attendees come up with their own parenting questions instead.
- A variation on the above variation: quiz mom with the questions and have the author of each question donate a quarter to the baby's first piggy bank for each question mom is able to answer.
- Have mom and dad alternate reading the Q&A to each other.

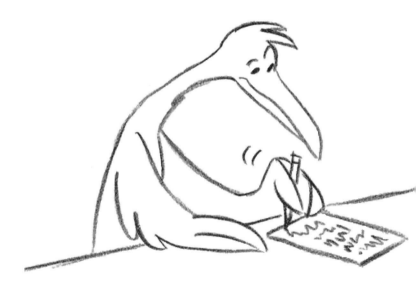

MEMORY/WORD GAMES

BABYING MOM

Remembering mom as a babe.

When
before/after baby is born

How
Ask mom to reveal a bunch of baby trivia about herself. These toddler tidbits might include:

- How many pounds did she weigh as a newborn?
- What was another name her parents wanted to name her?
- What was her favorite toy as a baby?
- Was she born by Cesarean section?
- What did she want to be when she was a toddler?
- What was her favorite food or toy?
- What did she call her blanket/pacifier?
- What animal was her childhood pet?
- What did she refuse to eat as a baby?

Make copies of your question list and pass out among guests to fill out. Have mom give the correct answers (and accompanying anecdote if applicable). The person with the mother lode of correct matches wins the game.

Variation/Tips
- If mom-to-be can't remember some of her baby facts, consult her mom.
- This variation engages all your guests. Have everyone write a tidbit of trivia about themselves as a baby on a scrap of paper. Collect the bits of trivia and have guests randomly draw a piece. Each person reads their trivia aloud and guesses who wrote it.

BABY SITTING

A test of observation skills.

When

before/after baby is born

How

Have an array of small baby-related things on hand, such as a bib, rattle, sock, diaper, bottle, baby powder, formula, etc. As guests arrive, give each person an infant item. Arrivals have to wear this item; pass out ribbon—bulky items can be hung around their neck, or tied to their waist, strapped to their back, etc. They will baby-sit the thing until you're ready to explain how to play the game.

Let mingling go on for about five to ten minutes. Then announce the game's start by asking for the return of all the wee wear. Arrange these baby basics out in front of the group. Distribute pen and paper. They now have five minutes to recall who was wearing what baby item. Your most accurate observer takes a prize.

Variation/Tips

❑ If there are a lot of baby items, write a unique number in front of each item on the table. This way, guests can simply write a name next to a number on their list.

❑ If the guest list is so large that it's impractical to buy an item for each participant, an alternative is to simply write the name of a baby item on a name-tag for each guest to wear.

❑ Or, require people to take on the name of the item they're given. All attendees have to address each other by their assigned baby item, such as "Hey, Baby Powder!", instead of their actual name. If an actual name is used, the person who was incorrectly addressed gets to take the name caller's baby item as a penalty. Whoever has the most items collected in the end wins. You can maintain this game throughout the entire party, or limit it to a half hour's play.

THE FAMILY NAME

Three's a crowd, but what do you call a bunch of geese?

When
before/after baby is born

How
This tests your ability to name groups of animals. Examples: a *herd* of cattle, a *pod* or *school* of whales. Read off a type of creature and your pack should yell out answers. The individual with the first correct answer gets a penny; collect the most pennies to win.

Creature	Grouping	Creature	Grouping
ants	army/colony	horses	herd/drove
bees	hive/swarm	hummingbirds	charm
cats	cluster/clutter	jellyfish	smack/fluther
crows	murder	kangaroos	mob/troop
dogs	pack	lions	pride/troop
ducks	team/paddling	moles	labor
elephants	herd/parade	monkeys	barrel/tribe
ferrets	business	owls	parliament/stare
fish	school/catch	parrots	flock/company
frogs	army/colony	rabbits	colony/bury
geese	gaggle/skein	swallows	gulp
grasshoppers	cloud	storks	mustering

Variation/Tips
❑ Easier way to play: display the group names in alphabetical order for players to choose from. See Appendix for more groupings.
❑ Or, play this like Memory. Make a set of cards with all the animals written on them and another set with all the group names. Mix up each set of cards, place each card word side down on a table. Players take turns flipping over one card from each set. If they get a match, they keep the set of cards, if not, turn them back over. Whoever has the most cards in the end wins.

THE FUNNIES

Identifying cartoons that are out of character.

When
before/after baby is born

How
To prepare for this game, cut out a frame from a variety of Sunday comic strips and tape each frame to a piece of blank paper. You'll want to have about ten different frames, from old favorites as well as newer serials. Write the title of each comic the frame was taken from on the back of the page.

Display the cartoons. Your comic marvels try to identify the title of each comic strip by writing down their guesses on a piece of paper. Read off the answers, the most correct matches out of this cartoon commune wins.

Variation/Tips
❑ A variation is to have comic contenders recall the name of the character in addition to the comic title.
❑ To make the game harder, cut out just the comic's main character and a bubble of dialog.

KIDDING AROUND

Show and tell pint-sized achievements.

When
before/after baby is born

How
This is ideal for smaller groups. Individuals write down a brief description of an achievement from their childhood (such as placing first in a spelling bee or how a scout badge was earned) on a piece of paper. The kid kudos can be something awe-inspiring or giggle-inducing or just plain cute. Your memory makers have to keep it under five sentences and not write their names. Collect the papers.

Randomly pick a paper one at a time and read out loud each tyke triumph. The gang decides whose success story they've heard. Once an answer is settled on, the true achievement author reveals him/herself.

Variation/Tips
❑ Spread the good news around, let players take turns randomly drawing papers to read out loud to the gathering.
❑ To make the game more competitive, players write who they think is behind each accomplishment on another piece of paper. After you've gone through all the tyke triumphs, go through them again and ask the author to identify him/herself. Person who correctly ID's the most feats wins.
❑ You don't have to limit these memories to an achievement, expand the topic to rowdy rebellion or funny feat or any unique childhood experience.

MATERNITY LEAVE

Armchair globetrotting from here to maternity.

When
before/after baby is born

How
Day trippers take turns calling out a unique city, state, or country. The only rule is that the destination has to start with the letter of the alphabet that the previous locale ended in.

For example, the first traveler says "New York," the next voyager has to think of a city, state or country that starts with the letter "K," such as "Kansas." The following player has to name a place that starts with "S," like "Singapore" and so on. Sightseers get the heave-ho when they make a roundtrip (name a city, state or country that's been announced already) or can't call out the next locale. The last jet-setter remaining is your geographic genius.

Variation/Tips
❏ Have someone who doesn't have wanderlust sit out and write down the cities, states, and countries as they're named so that any duplicates can be caught more easily.

MEETING OF THE MINDS

Think of what mother knows best.

When
before/after baby is born

How
Create a list of ten baby-related words. For example: apple, baby, cotton, blanket, diaper, crib, night light, saltines, formula, bootie. Distribute pencil and paper to players. Read off the items one at a time. Everybody, including mom, writes down the first word that comes to mind after hearing the baby word read to them. Players may not share or discuss their answers.

Once you've finished going through the list, reveal the true purpose of the game: to determine who thinks just like mom. For example, mom might write "sauce" in response to "apple," whoever else responded in kind gets a point. Mom continues reading off her answers for comparison. Get the most matches to win.

Variation/Tips
❏   If there are no matches per word, bend the rule so that anyone who has written any of mom's reaction words gets a point per match.
❏   This version has everyone, including mom, write a list of all the baby items they can think of in three minutes. Then mom reads off her list and players circle the items they've written that match the items from mom's list. Player with the most matches thinks like a mom.
❏   A twist on this match game: ask dad-to-be or grandma-to-be to make up the list that players have to try to match.
❏   Or, create a game sheet of things dad could have said and actually said when he learned mom was pregnant. Guests have to try to circle the remarks that dad actually made from a list of possible comments.

A corny tale for the apple of mom's eye.

When
before/after baby is born

How
Players veg out by writing a note to the baby, incorporating as many fruit and vegetable words as possible within 5 minutes. For example, "Orange you glad that your mom and dad have gone Bananas creating a Peachy-keen nursery room for you?"

Authors take turns harvesting their veggie tales by reading them to the group. Award an apple to the writer of the most bountiful story (uses the most fruit and vegetable references) or most popular among the group by a show of hands.

Variation/Tips
❑ Team players into pairs and give them 10 minutes to craft a more fruitful fantasy.
❑ An easier variation starts with a pre-written story that has the fruit and vegetable words missing for players to fill in. See the Appendix for the Producing A Great Baby story for an example. Type up the story without the fruit/vegetable words and make copies for your guests to fill-in the blanks. After everybody has written in their answers, read the complete story to let them check their story against yours.
❑ For this variation, give each player a carrot. Randomly select one to hold a candy bar instead of a carrot. Players continuously pass the item in their hand while mom reads the Producing a Great Baby story (in the Appendix) out loud. Guests simultaneously and continuously pass the item in the same direction, but every time they hear a fruit or vegetable, the passing direction changes and goes the opposite way. Whoever ends up with the candy bar in hand at the end of the story wins.

MULTILINGUAL BABY

It's still a baby by any other name.

When
before/after baby is born

How
Most languages call a baby a baby, or easily recognizable variation:
Bebe (Spanish), or Bambino (Italian). This game involves identifying
the language based on its version of the word "infant." The left
column below lists "infant" in different languages. All the languages
represented here are in the right column.

1.	kind	Dutch
2.	nourrisson	French
3.	zuigeling	German
4.	infante	Hawaiian
5.	nino	Italian
6.	spedbarn	Lithuanian
7.	mladenec	Norwegian
8.	sanggol	Russian
9.	eifele	Spanish
10.	bebek	Tagalog
11.	pepe	Turkish
12.	kudikis	Yiddish

Print a copy for each guest. Your linguists draw a line between the
"infant" and matching language. Most correct matches wins.

Variation/Tips

❑ Answers: 1. German, 2, French, 3. Dutch, 4. Italian, 5. Spanish, 6.
Norwegian, 7. Russian, 8. Tagalog, 9. Yiddish, 10. Turkish, 11.
Hawaiian, 12. Lithuanian.

❑ Instead of using the word "infant," try multilingual variations on
"daddy" or "mommy."

NAME CALLING

Player who drops the most names wins.

When
before/after baby is born

How
Give each player a pen and paper. Spell out the full name of mom and dad for players to write down as reference. Using only the letters from these two names, guests must create as many first names for the baby (boy and girl) as they can. For example, if there are three A's between the two names, then the letter A can be used up to three times to create a new name. Give players five minutes to be creative and make a name for themselves.

Name callers take turns reading off the monikers they've created. Everyone else listens closely and must cross off the name on their list if at least one other player has the same name. In other words, a name only counts if no one else has thought of it. From the ones that remain, mom picks the name she likes most or judges most unique and awards a prize to the player most worthy of the name.

Variation/Tips
❑ Have a baby name book on hand to referee any challenges that arise.
❑ Another way to play: declare the person who names the most names the winner. However, set down some ground rules so that creative types are not just writing down nonsense words for names. A name counts only if the group agrees that it's a name or if it's a unique spelling of an existing name.
❑ Ask everyone to write down only names ending with y, my, ie, an, or nie, etc. or names starting with am, ch, ca, ba, or sh, etc.
❑ Baby's name is already decided upon? Play this variation instead: have players make as many baby-related words (that are three letters or more) as they can out of the baby's full name.

NEWS FLASH

Telegraph a funny message from baby words.

When
before/after baby is born

How
First, you'll need a list of six words like diaper, powder, crib, rattle, burp, wipes (or create your own). Give players paper and pen.

Read off the first word on your list, "diaper" and players should write down the word "diaper," on their paper. Players treat DIAPER like an acronym and write a telegram where each letter of the word dictates another word. For example, DIAPER could be "Did Ian At Princeton Eat Radish?"

Give word smiths one minute to compose as unique or thoughtful or funny a sentence as they can. Then read off the next word on the list and continue until finished with the war of words. People take turns reading their baby-grams and signal for their favorite wire with applause.

Variation/Tips
❑ Use the baby's name for inspiration instead. Let's say baby's name is MARY. The cable crafters write advice for growing up, and each word in the sentence has to begin with a letter in the name like this: Make A Ravishing Year.
❑ Or, challenge players to write a sentence for each letter in baby's (or mom's) name, each sentence has to start with a letter in baby's name. For example: Mary, this advice is for you. Always be nice to your siblings. Really try to live life to the fullest. Yearn to be the best at everything you do. Encourage your players to be creative in their writing, suggest they try to theme the sentences around advice for the parent or child.

OLD WIVES' TALES

Put baby gender prediction myths to the test.

When
before baby is born

How
Attendees take turns asking mom the questions below, her answers are supposed to predict the sex of her baby. (These questions are based on old wives' tales.) Circle mom's answer under the appropriate column. When finished, tally up the total. The predicted gender will be the column with the most answers circled.

	Boy	Girl
Do you crave...	Sour	Sweet
Do you crave the heel of a loaf of bread?	Yes	No
Are you drinking orange juice....	Less	More
Is the baby's position....	High	Low
The shape of your stomach looks like a...	Basketball	Watermelon
Baby kicks this most often...	Ribs	Stomach
What side does baby kick most often?	Right	Left
How does baby react to music?	Holds still	Dances
Do you know baby's heart rate?	<139	>140
Is mom smiling more?	Yes	No
Ask mom to show us her hands.	Palms Down	Palms Up
Ask mom to stare in the mirror for a minute, do her eyes dilate?	Yes	No
Does your hair feel shiny and full bodied or thinner and stringier?	Full	Thin
Do your hands feel...	Rough	Smooth
Are your fingernails growing...	Faster	Same
Hair on legs growing faster?	Yes	No
Do your legs seem to be growing larger?	Yes	No
Any weight gain on the backside?	None	Some
Does your face feel...	Same	Fuller
Do your feet feel...	Colder	Same
What color is maternal grandma's hair?	Gray	Other

	Boy	Girl
Do you sleep with your head to the....	North	South
Do you feel more sleepy or less?	Less	More
What side do you prefer to sleep on?	Left	Right
Any dreams of a boy or girl?	Boy	Girl
Are you having severe morning sickness?	No	Yes
Is your breathing free & easy or is there shortness of breath?	Short	Free
How's your overall feeling?	Comfy	Not Comfy
Does your kitchen seem busier?	Yes	No
Does mom pick up a coffee cup by the...	Handle	Sides
What date was the baby conceived?	Odd	Even
On the night of conception, was the moon...	Partial	Full
What kind of underwear does dad wear?	Briefs	Boxers
Does Dad feel...	Relaxed	Nervous
Is dad getting more household projects done?	Yes	No
Has dad's weight changed?	Gain	Same
Dangle a threaded needle by its string over mom's tummy, does it...	Swing	Circles

Variation/Tips

❑ If mom doesn't know the answer to specific questions, just skip them. Also, don't feel you have to go through the entire list.

❑ Make a quiz of old wives' tales. On top of the game sheet write "Will mom have a boy or girl if she..." and list symptoms like this: is craving more sweets? is smiling more? conceived the baby in a full moon? Players write their answer of Boy or Girl per question.

❑ With the quiz version, pit players head to head on ten questions at a time to see who gets the most correct. Play additional questions for another set of players. You can also pit mom vs. dad, or mom vs. her mom, mom vs. her best friend, etc.

❑ Different variations of these folk wisdoms are in constant circulation, adjust the game sheet as desired or add your own.

❑ Even if mom already knows the baby's sex, this questionnaire is still a fun way to see how the results compare.

PARTS OF A WHOLE

A baby anatomy lesson.

When

before/after baby is born

How

Name the body part that fills out a proverb. Most correct answers wins. Hand out copies of the sample quiz below or foot your own.

1. Beauty is only ? deep.
2. A bird in ? is worth two in the bush.
3. Now the shoe is on the other ?.
4. Don't let the grass grow under your ?.
5. Turn the other ?.
6. Absence makes the ? grow fonder.
7. What the ? doesn't see, the ? doesn't grieve over.
8. Never look a gift horse in the ?.
9. Sticks and stones may break my ? but words will never hurt me.
10. A way to a man's ? is through his ?.
11. Don't cut your ? off to spite your ?.
12. Many ? make light work.

Variation/Tips

❑ Answers: 1. skin, 2. hand, 3. foot, 4. feet, 5. cheek, 6. heart, 7. eye, heart, 8. mouth, 9. bones, 10. heart, stomach, 11. nose, face, 12. hands.

❑ Reverse play: Name the body part and have guests write a proverb containing that specific body part.

❑ Challenge players to name baby parts that are also parts of something nonliving. For example, a baby has an arm and so does a chair. More combos: comb = teeth, macaroni = elbow, potato = eyes, orange = navel, clock = hands, shoe = heel, onion = skin, etc.

❑ Name body parts that are only made up of three letter words. The answers: arm, eye, ear, gum, hip, jaw, leg, lip, lid, rib, toe.

PETTING ZOO

Identify stuffed animals by touch.

When
before/after baby is born

How
You'll need five different stuffed animals, like a bear, dog, giraffe, fish, and monkey. Put each animal in an empty pillowcase.

Assemble players into a circle for this funny farm. Pass out the bagged animals, warning players that they're not allowed to look inside the pillowcases. The object is to identify the animal inside each bag after petting it.

One person holds a pillowcase for the player on their left to reach in and feel the animal inside. Players pass the pillowcase to their right and continue with play. Competitors have to remember all the animals they petted.

After the animal assortment has made a round, collect the bags. Farm out a piece of paper and pencil to everyone so they can write down their five guesses. Then show the animals to the group. Player with the winning touch will have the correct animals listed in the correct order.

Variation/Tips
❑ Before playing with recently purchased animals, be sure to remove any tags on them.
❑ Forget reaching inside the pillowcase, have players identify each animal by touching them through the pillowcase and passing it on.
❑ Increase the number of animals to ten to increase the game's difficulty.
❑ Award the animals as prizes for this and other games, or give to mom to furnish her nursery.

PIECE OF CAKE

Sweetie pies compete for brownie points.

When
before/after baby is born

How
Serve up this calorie-free quiz to guests. Player with most correct answers takes the cake. Each answer must be unique (that is, the same kind of cake cannot be used more than once). Answers follow in the Variation/Tips.

1. What cake is eaten annually?
2. What cake bears fruit?
3. What cake is heavenly?
4. What cake is the biggest flop?
5. What is a mouse's favorite cake?
6. What cake is served in stacks in the morning?
7. What cake fits nicely on a saucer?
8. What cake is found on the ocean floor?
9. What cake will always go out with you?
10. What cake weighs the most?
11. What cake is on the dark side?
12. What cake should be eaten in bed?
13. What cake is a child's game?
14. What cake is always served frozen?
15. What kind of cake weighs diamonds?
16. What's a really dirty cake?
17. What's a midget cake?
18. What cake helps tie the knot?
19. What cake is well seasoned?
20. Name the cakes that aren't very cool.
21. What cake comes with a cup of joe?
22. What's the sexiest cake of all?

Variation/Tips

❑ The answers (note that some have more than one possible answer): 1: Birthday Cake, 2: Fruitcake, 3: Angel Food Cake, 4: Upside Down Cake, 5: Cheesecake, 6: Pancake, 7: Cupcake/Tea Cake, 8: Sponge Cake, 9: Date Cake/Hoecake, 10: Pound Cake, 11: Devil's Food Cake, 12: Sheet Cake, 13: Patty Cake, 14: Ice Cream Cake, 15: Carrot Cake, 16: Mud Cake, 17: Shortcake, 18: Wedding Cake, 19: Spice Cake, 20: Hotcakes, 21: Coffeecake, 22: Beefcake

❑ Let them eat cake after the quiz, everyone will have worked up an appetite for their just desserts.

❑ This variation conjures up baby names:
GIRLS: 1. A type of wine, 2. Fine wine glass, 3. A fragrant flower, 4. Christmastime berries and leaves, 5. Fourth month of the year, 6. Happiness, 7. To engage in a lawsuit, 8. Having trust, 9. The color of the beach, 10. Another way to call a cat, 11. Effortless beauty or charm, 12. Very small river.
BOYS: 1. Very honest, 2. Permit a privilege, 3. Unit of measurement, 4. Small whirlpool, 5. An invoice, 6. A blue-feathered bird, 7. One who searches for something, 8. A college faculty member, 9. A small cut, 10. A beam of light, 11. Fancy and exclusive, 12. Determination

Girls' Answers: 1. Brandy, 2. Crystal, 3. Rose or Lily, 4. Holly, 5. April, 6. Joy, 7. Sue, 8. Faith, 9. Sandy, 10. Kitty, 11. Grace, 12. Brooke.
Boys' Answers: 1. Frank, 2. Grant, 3. Graham, 4. Eddy, 5. Bill, 6. Jay, 7. Hunter, 8. Dean, 9. Nick, 10. Ray. 11. Tony. 12. Will

PINNED ON MOM

Let mom wear her sock on her sleeve.

When
before/after baby is born

How
You'll need to prepare some props before playing this game. Get an old bathrobe and a bunch of newborn necessities such as baby wipes, wash cloth, pacifier, rattle, cotton balls, tweezers, socks, bonnet, diaper, teething cookie, feeding spoon, teething ring, etc. Use safety pins to pin all these items all over the robe.

To play, mom wears this baby bathrobe and models it for her guests for one minute. Mom leaves the room to remove her robe. Give players pen and paper and three minutes to remember all the items pinned to her robe. When time's up, mom brings the garment back out to determine who remembered the most items.

Variation/Tips
❑   If some items are too difficult to pin, tie a piece of ribbon around the item and pin the ribbon to the robe.
❑   Instead of pinning goodies to a shirt, pile everything into a baby tub or hang on a clothesline. Briefly parade to guests before covering with a blanket.
❑   Or, pile everything into a pillowcase. Have guests reach into the pillowcase one at a time to feel out what's inside. Give each guest 30 seconds in the bag. Let them write down everything they can remember. The one who remembers the most items bags the win.
❑   Surprise your guests with this twist on the above, send mom out of the room with the robe/pillowcase and ask players to recall not the things they saw/felt, but what mom was wearing!
❑   Another variation: remove five items after viewing and bring the robe/pillowcase back out to see if anyone can remember all five of the missing items (or come closest).

POPULARITY CONTEST

Name each decade's most popular boy and girl.

When
before/after baby is born

How
Give players a paper and pen. The name of the game is to report the most popular boy and girl's name from each decade.

According to the Social Security Administration (www.ssa.gov), the most popular names for the following decades are:

1940: James, Mary
1950: John, Linda
1960: David, Mary
1970: Michael, Jennifer
1980: Michael, Jennifer
1990: Michael, Jessica
2000: Jacob, Emily

Name the player with the most correct answers the winner.

Variation/Tips
❑ This variation requires a little more prep work, but is more personalized to your guests. Pick a year of some significance to mom. Using that year, look up the names of all your invited guests to see what number each name placed in terms of popularity for that year. Give a copy of the guest list to all your players. They have to write the number where their name (and their fellow players) placed for the selected year. Most correct guesses to win.

RHYME AND REASON

Calling out childhood rhymes.

When
before/after baby is born

How
All you need is a book of nursery rhymes for the crowd, just randomly pick a rhyme line to read out loud. First player to shout out the title of the rhyme earns a point each time. Then continue pulling a dozen different stanzas for this rhyming bonanza. Score the most points to grin over your win.

Variation/Tips

❑ Or, provide just the beginning of a verse and challenge guests to finish the rest of the line.

❑ Write silly summaries of famous nursery rhymes and have players identify the rhyme. Some examples: Visually impaired vermin marathon; The story of the accidental omelet; Inept coed water-fetchers, Naturally luminous body in the night sky. The answers: Three Blind Mice, Humpty Dumpty, Jack and Jill, Twinkle, Twinkle Little Star.

❑ A version for visual thinkers. Display a prop from each rhyme to see if guests can name the rhyme it's from. For example, you might have a pair of dark glasses, an empty egg shell, a pail, and a cut-out in the shape of a star (the answers are the same as the last variation).

❑ Pull lines from popular children's nursery rhymes, but make some subtle changes to them. For example: Mary had a little dog, its fur was white as snow. Type up and copy the modified rhymes. Distribute to guests who then have to fix the rhymes.

❑ This variation is a nice conversation starter. Ask guests to bring their favorite baby book to the shower to fill baby's first library. Allow your bookworms to speak briefly about the book they brought if they want to.

SWEET EXPECTATIONS

Sweet talking the pregnancy.

When
before/after baby is born

How
This is played like Memory. Players flip over a pregnancy related card and a candy card in hopes of getting a match. For example, a correct match would be College Fund and 100 Grand. Player who finds a matching pair removes the cards and wins that piece of candy. If the cards don't match, flip them back over. Below is a list of the correct pairings (or create your own). Write each item separately onto individual index cards:

Contractions : Whoppers
Little girl : Baby Ruth
Baby's father : Big Hunk
Epidural : Lifesavers
Breast feeding : Milky Way
Baby fat : Chunky
Hospital bills : Pay Day
Triplets : Three Musketeers
Lullaby : Symphony

Labor : Rocky Road
Little boys : Mike & Ike
Conception : Skor
Twins : Twix
Umbilical cord : Twizzlers
College fund : 100 Grand
Dirty diaper : Milk Duds
Postpartum tummy : Jelly Belly
Loving Parents : Kisses

Mix up your cards and set them word side down. Players take turns flipping over two cards at a time. Whether there's a match or not, play proceeds to the next player. Award candy as matches are made.

Variation/Tips
❏ Or, list all the pregnancy words in one column and candy in another on a game sheet. Attendees draw lines between pairs.
❏ Display all these candies and let guests write stories using as many of the sweets as possible. Example: Jane was feeling Chunky until she realized she was pregnant with Baby Ruth...

TAKING NAMES

Sleuthing the meaning of names.

When

before/after baby is born

How

A bit of prep work is required beforehand, but this look at what makes a name results in great conversation later. When you've assembled your final guest list, look up the meaning of each first name in a baby name book (or on the internet). Create a game sheet by writing a brief summary of name meanings in one column, and then randomly list the first names on a second column. Make as many copies of your game sheet as you have attendees.

To play, everybody tries to match a moniker with its meaning on their game sheet by drawing a line between pairs. Once everybody is finished, read aloud the correct meanings to each name so players can check their answers. Lavish praise on your big name winner.

Variation/Tips

❏ Instead of matching a name to its meaning, match it to the etymology (origin), (see Appendix).

❏ Or, type up the name meanings on individual name badges. Give each guest a badge with their own name on it and a randomly selected name meaning badge. Charge guests with calling on the person who has their name meaning.

❏ Don't limit yourself to the names of your attendees on your game sheet, include some unique names or names with interesting backgrounds.

❏ This version is the simplest to play. Have players take turns telling the story (there's always a story) behind their name (or nickname).

WE'RE IN THE MONEY

When money talks, it says baby's name.

When
before/after baby is born

How
Everyone needs a pencil and dollar bill to make this run for the money. Announce the names that mom has chosen for the different sexes for her little dividend, such as "Heather" if it's a girl and "Robbie" if it's a boy. And spell out the names.

The first money manager to find and circle all the letters in both names on their bill wins the game. There are many letters on the front and back of the bill. The only rule is that letters can be used only once (for example, two different "e's" should be circled to spell Heather). Since time is money, tell everybody to start circling!

Variation/Tips
❏ While the dollar bill has most letters of the alphabet, it doesn't have all of them. Check beforehand that both names can be found on the bill. (See more about this in the last variation.)

❏ If the baby's name hasn't been decided on, have people seek out mom and/or dad's names or the names of any other special person in baby's life, such as grandma or grandpa.

❏ Another twist on this money madness: players race to be the first person to circle all the letters of their own first and last name on the bill. Depending on the series of the bill, the signatures will vary, meaning it's possible to find some letters (such as "J") on one bill and not others. Suggest to players they might want to empty their pockets or pass the buck to find the bill with the letter they need.

WHISPERING SWEET NOTHINGS

Share sugar and spice and everything nice with mom.

When
before/after baby is born

How
You'll need the following candies all mixed together in a bowl: pillow mints, gummy bears, chocolate covered nuts, and cinnamon candy.

Pass the bowl around to attendees, they pick only one piece of candy. When everyone has a treat in hand, read the instructions below to the gathering.

The candy you've chosen dictates the kind of sweet talk you will give mom:

Mint. Great advice is worth a mint. So give mom a useful parenting hint.
Gummy bear. Like mom, these candies are sweet and fair. Share a nice story about her to show you care.
Chocolate. Women go nuts for chocolate, it's no secret, name some treats a child will target.
Cinnamon Candy. Romance tends to be forgotten when raising a tot. Share some advice to keep the marriage red hot.

Go around the room. After the candy call, let every sweet tooth indulge in their favorite treat.

Variation/Tips
❑ The organizer of this game should go first to give an example and give the group time to formulate their advice.
❑ If you need a substitute for chocolate covered nuts, use any candy that has chocolate in it (like miniature chocolate bars).

WORD TO THE WISE

Wise up by completing proverbs.

When
before/after baby is born

How
Print up a list of popular (and less common) adages on pieces of paper. You'll need one proverb for every two guests attending. Cut out each sentence individually, then in half so that the beginning of the proverb is on one piece of paper and the other half is on the other piece of paper. For example: "An ounce of prevention" and "is worth a pound of cure." make up a pair. Put all the proverb halves in a paper bag and mix well.

Have every wise guy and gal draw a piece of paper. Once everybody has a proverb piece, have them mingle to locate the other half of the proverb. When everybody is paired up, they read off the proverb they've created to see if they got it right.

Variation/Tips
❏ More proverbs you can use: A bird in the hand is worth two in the bush. A fair-weather friend changes with the wind. Birds of a feather flock together. Children and fools speak the truth. Empty wagons make the most noise. Don't cut off your nose to spite your face. Great oaks from little acorns grow. Hope is a good breakfast, but a bad supper. It is easier to give good counsel than to follow it. Look for dirt, and you'll find it. Money is a good servant, but a bad master. To err is human, to forgive is divine. Whatever is worth doing, is worth doing well. You will catch more flies with honey than with vinegar.
❏ Another way to play: create a game sheet of incomplete proverbs and let guests fill in the sentences. Then read the answers and reward the wise one with the most correctly filled out proverbs.

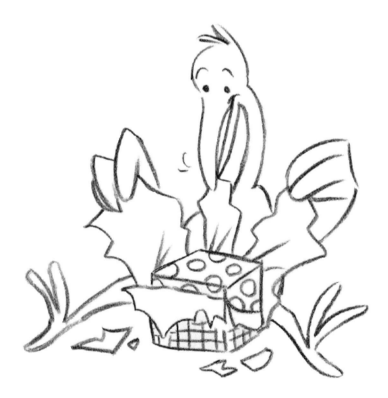

ACTIVE GAMES

BARNYARD CRITTERS

Mew, chirp, or baa your way to your peeps.

When
before/after baby is born

How
Before the party prep: write down a type of animal on two pieces of paper (so that you'll have two papers sporting each kind of animal). So, if you have 16 guests, you'll need 8 farm critters: duck, sheep, dog, cat, goat, horse, chicken, pig. If you have more than 16 guests attending or you have an odd number of attendees, duplicate some of the animals (it's OK to have 4 horses, 2 pigs, and 3 chickens, or any combination you please). Fold up the papers and put in a bag.

To play, randomly farm out slips of paper to each person. Warn them not to chicken out by revealing their animal identity yet. Tell your players straight from the horse's mouth that they are now the baby animal written on their paper and the goal is to find another baby of the same species on the farm. Since the cat's got their tongue, they can only "talk" with each other as the animal they've been assigned. In other words, ducks should quack and horses should neigh. Put a time limit of three minutes to prevent the gab session from running until the cows come home.

Variation/Tips
- This is a great ice-breaking game, play it early in the gathering.
- Everybody wins in this game. Once the animal whisperers have been paired up, you can use these groupings to play other games.

COPYCAT

Sleuth out the original from the imitators.

When
before/after baby is born

How
Pick one player to be a Mouse and send out of the room for one minute. The rest gather into a circle and select someone to be the Cat. The Cat leads the copycats in making any gesture or movement in place. For example, if the Cat waves, the rest of the group waves also. Everybody keeps waving until the Cat does something else like laugh, then everybody else laughs.

While this is going on, the Mouse comes in and tries to sort the Cat from the copycats. Mouse gets only three attempts to correctly locate the leader. The Cat must perform at least three different movements before the Mouse's three guesses are up. Whoever succeeds first is the cat's meow.

Variation/Tips
❑ Other things the leader might do: wink, flap arms, waggle finger, tap foot, clap hands, smack lips, etc.
❑ To make the game of cat and mouse harder, designate two Mice who race to be the first to locate the Cat. Play several rounds and change the Cat and Mouse roles with each round.
❑ Instead of standing around in a circle, have players stand in random parts of the room and wander around during the game.

DATING

A different kind of dating game.

When
before/after baby is born

How
This cute activity helps to break the ice and encourage mingling early in the gathering. Have everyone write just the month and date of their birth on a scrap of paper—not year. Gather these scraps in a bag, shake it up, and let guests draw a scrap. When everybody has a piece of paper in hand, send them off to locate and introduce themselves to their "date."

Once everybody is up to date (reunited with their correct birth date), announce the baby's due date and award a prize to the person whose birth date is closest.

Variation/Tips
❑   Or, just to be different, award a prize to the person whose birth date is farthest from the expected due date.

DIAPER SERVICE

A diaper tossing contest.

When
before/after baby is born

How
Play this waste management game outside. You'll need ten disposable diapers and a diaper pail. Pour about half a cup of water into each diaper and pile into a bowl. Set the diaper pail about 10 feet away from the bowl.

Diaper disposers take turns tossing the wet waste one at a time into the pail. Record the number of successful slam dunks per player. Play continues until everyone's had a turn. Whoever successfully trashes the most wet diapers scores!

Variation/Tips
❑ If you don't have a pail of any kind, just about any container can be substituted—the smaller the opening, the more difficult the game. You may want to weigh down the container with some rocks to prevent it from tipping.

❑ If you have a tie and players aren't pooped out, run a play-off round with the diaper pail 15 feet away from the bowl.

DIAPER TAG

Sniff out the diaper that missed the call of nature.

When
before/after baby is born

How
Before the party, you'll need as many square white napkins and safety pins as you have guests. Lightly smear some chocolate syrup or mustard in the center of each napkin except for one—leave that clean. Individually fold each napkin into an upside down triangle, then fold the bottom point up to the top of the fold. Fold both left and right corners to the middle of the fold. Pin closed with a safety pin and set aside on a plate.

As guests arrive, let them pick a diaper and write their name on the diaper, then wear it as a name tag. At the desired time, everybody opens their diapers. Person with the clean diaper comes up smelling like roses!

Variation/Tips
- Play the reverse: make most of them clean. Don't pooh-pooh whoever finds the dirty diaper, they're the winner.
- To seal each diaper, melt some household wax and dip each napkin diaper into the wax to cover. Let dry on wax paper before using.
- Another way to play is to insert a small white mint candy into each diaper, substituting a small colored mint into one diaper. Proceed as usual, whoever gets the colored mint has the poopie. Other variations include white/dark chocolate or white/black raisins, etc.
- If mom's expecting twins, put in two of each mint.
- Dislike donning diaper couture? Set a bowl of them (make double or triple the number of guests) in the center of the room. At the words "Dirty diapers!" everybody tries to find the one clean diaper, but they may only grab one and open one at a time.

A little game of airplane.

When
before/after baby is born

How
Give guests a taste of the struggle to feed another mouth with this game. Turn an empty shoe box or tissue box on its side so that it stands up the tall way. Draw in eyes and nose, then cut out an oval for the mouth that's about two inches (or length of your pinky finger) tall and wide. Embellish with a bib and cap if you wish. Fill a big bowl with a bag of cotton balls, you'll also need a big spoon.

Players take turns spoon feeding as many cotton balls as possible to the baby within one minute—while blindfolded. Whoever stuffs the baby's face with the most cotton balls during the spoon sprint wins.

Variation/Tips
❑ The wider the mouth opening, the easier the game is for your players. Have someone hold the baby still during the feeding.
❑ If you have a silver spoon on hand, use it for this game!
❑ A whole new ballgame: apply petroleum jelly to player's nose; they transfer as many cotton balls as they can from one plate to another (just an inch away) by pressing their nose into the cotton and shaking them loose (no hands). Give a time-limit of a minute per player. Transfer the most balls to win.
❑ A variation on the above, provide just one big empty bowl on a table, scatter a bunch of cotton balls on the table. Whoever gets the most balls into the bowl with their jelly covered nose is the winner. (They can't use their hands.)
❑ Or, blindfold a player and give the player a big serving spoon (the heavier the better), she has one minute to transfer as many cotton balls to another bowl as possible. Again, player who transfers the most balls is winner.

FOOD GROUPS

See who can stomach this balanced taste-test.

When
before/after baby is born

How
Buy seven jars of different flavored baby food (try to have each food group represented: dairy, meat, vegetable, fruit, and bread or grains). You'll also need a box of wooden sticks. Cover the label of each baby food jar with paper, number the jar. Write up a master key of the baby jars for reference. Pass one baby food jar around at a time. Taste testers use a new stick to dip into each baby food jar. After digesting each flavor, they write the food group it belongs to. Player with the most correct answers can savor the taste of victory.

Variation/Tips
❑ Have another bite: challenge players to identify the food itself.
❑ Check that players don't have any food allergies or sensitivities.
❑ For those who have a taste for it, get five players to compete to see who can chug their jar of baby food the fastest.
❑ Discard any leftover baby food after the game.
❑ Baby food is too hard to swallow? Have players identify the food jars by looks (and/or smell) only. Another variation of this game is to pair similar looking baby food jars together without their labels (applesauce and pears; carrots and squash). Label each jar a letter of the alphabet. Create a master list of all the baby food you have, plus a few that aren't in there. Copy this list and give one to each player, players try to differentiate the similar looking food pairs based on the list of foods provided by sight.
❑ Or, try to guess the flavor of a variety of juices instead. All kids love juice right? This game is much easier to execute if you purchase and use disposable mini-cups so that players don't have to rinse out cups in between sips. Provide each taster with a couple tablespoons of each liquid.

Paint a pretty picture among neighbors.

When
before/after baby is born

How
Form a neighborhood by sitting everyone in a circle one arm length apart. Give each good neighbor a piece of paper and pen. Tell players to be neighborly by greeting their neighbor on their left and right.

This is a test to see how quickly news travels in the neighborhood. Before the game, hand draw a picture of a baby being delivered by a stork to a house. Show this piece of news to one player in the circle for only 5 seconds. This player then has to draw the news she saw on her piece of paper from memory and show her drawing to her neighbor on her right. This second player also has 5 seconds to view this new drawing, then pass the news to their neighbor and so on until the news has traveled through the entire neighborhood (go one round in counter-clockwise direction).

Compare the end drawing with the start drawing to see how the news made it through the grapevine. It'll be a hoot.

Variation/Tips
❏   Put a time limit of 30 seconds on drawing each image to keep the news moving.
❏   To prevent cheating, tell the neighborhood they can only look at their neighbor's picture when it is their turn to draw.
❏   Ideas for other messages to pass around: having won the lottery, announcing the completion of a home theater room, an invitation to a baby shower... use your imagination or randomly select a player to make up a message to relay. The more complex the idea, the more likely it will get garbled in transmission.

HANDYMAN

Single-handedly clean up for the win.

When
before/after baby is born

How
Spread out a variety of kitchen utensils on a table. These utensils can include tongs, serving spoons and forks, ladles, spatulas, whisks, measuring cups and spoons, hand graters, potato/garlic masher, egg timer, mushroom scrubber, etc.

Players take turns trying to pick up as many utensils they can with only one hand. Their turn ends when they drop an item. Get a handle on the most utensils to be crowned an iron chef.

Variation/Tips
❑ Don't use knives!
❑ Increase this pick-up game's difficulty by specifying four items that a player must grab before handling anything else.
❑ A variation that requires less props: clip a bunch of clothespins onto a plastic clothes hanger. A player uses one hand to hold the hanger and their other hand to remove and hold clothespins. Anytime the player drops a pin, their turn ends. The pinhead who single-handedly clutches the most pins wins.

HEN PARTY

Catch a rooster before it barnstorms the entire hen house.

When
before/after baby is born

How
Form the hen house by standing everyone in a circle, elect one to be the Farmer. Send the Farmer out of the room for one minute.

The remaining players are now all chickens. Give your chicks an egg to hold behind their back. Select one player to be a Rooster. The Rooster's job is to discreetly wink at any hen in the circle (while pretending to be a hen). Whoever the Rooster winks at must loudly bawk, bawk, bawk like a chicken and lay their egg in front of them. The Rooster doesn't start working until the Farmer comes back in.

Tell your Farmer that a Rooster has snuck into the hen house and his/her job is to observe and root out the Rooster before all the hens lay their eggs. However, the Farmer is only allowed to make three guesses. (The Rooster cannot "tag" the same hen twice.) This is essentially a race between the Farmer and Rooster. Allow the winner ample time to crow their victory.

Variation/Tips
- Encourage chickens to ham up their roles, but remind hens to discreetly maintain eye contact with the rooster.
- Depending on how big the farm is, the Farmer may elect to patrol inside or outside the circle during the game.
- If your players are game, you can play additional rounds using different Farmers and Roosters. Or for a faster paced game, select two Roosters and two Farmers.
- In place of using real eggs, you can substitute plastic ones.
- This game can be played sitting down.

ICE CREAM SCOOPER

A lickety-split contest to get the scoop.

When
before/after baby is born

How
Get the scoop before the party by making two paper ice cream cones. Take a sheet of 8.5" X 11" paper (or use brown construction paper) and roll it so that it looks like a big ice cream cone (use tape to affix). You'll also need a big bag of cotton balls and two ice cream scoops to dish up this race.

Pour the cotton balls into a big bowl. Call up two players to compete for the title of Big Dipper. Give each a paper ice cream cone and scoop. The object of the game is to get as many scoops of ice cream (the cotton balls) into their cones within two minutes. But before the super scoopers start, blindfold them. Now go!!

Variation/Tips
❑ For a double-dip of fun, call up pairs of players to compete against one another. Try competing pairs like sister vs. sister, mom vs. mom-in-law, or husband/boyfriend vs. wife/girlfriend, etc.

❑ Try to save empty gallon containers of ice cream before the gathering. After cleaning and drying it, use the container to store the cotton balls instead of a bowl.

LENDING A HAND

A creative way to lend a hand to the parents.

When
before/after baby is born

How
Everyone knows how much mom (and dad) can use a hand when the new baby comes. Send mom out of the room while guests trace their handprint on a colored piece of paper and cut out with scissors.

Everybody places their cut-out hand in one bag and forms a line. Mom has to match each hand print to the guest, by handing it over to that guest (don't tell her if she's right or wrong). When she's matched up all the hands, guests who were given the wrong hand should take a step backward. Let mom try one more hand-picked round if needed.

Variation/Tips
❑ If dad wants to play too, have mom and dad take turns talking to the hand and matching it.

❑ If the baby has arrived, have guests write a flattering adjective (intelligent, cute, etc.) describing the baby. Save the hand-outs for decorating baby's nursery, or make a mobile out of them.

❑ Here's another way to play: players write a coupon for a favor, i.e., worth one night's baby sitting, one home cooked meal, a new baby storybook, a cup of coffee for the parents, a CD of lullaby music (whatever a guest feels comfortable contributing) on their hand cut-out. Whatever hands are successfully matched are returned to the parents to redeem at their discretion.

❑ This variation is a nice way to give something back to guests. You'll need as many fresh flowers on stems as you have guests. Tie a foot-long section of 1" wide ribbon on each flower. As guests arrive, give them a flower and ask them to write some parenting advice on the ribbon. Collect the ribbons and read each aloud, players try to guess the author behind the advice.

LIKE TAKING CANDY FROM A BABY

Steady hands can steal the show.

When
before/after baby is born

How
The goal is to remove as much flour as you can from a mound without toppling the cereal balanced on top. You'll need a small coffee cup, flour, paper plates, tablespoons, and some square shaped cereal. Tightly pack the cup with flour, cover the top with a paper plate. While holding the plate against the cup, quickly turn the cup over, set the plate onto a table. Remove the cup, the flour holds the cup shape. Carefully center a square of cereal on top of the flour mound. Make as many of these mounds as you have players who want to play. Give each player an extra paper plate and a tablespoon.

Players use their spoon to take as much candy (the flour) away without the baby knowing it. (Players use the spare paper plate they've been given to hold the flour they remove.) Once the cereal falls off the mound, the thief is considered caught and stops. Once everybody's been caught by their baby, measure the removed flour to determine who parted the most candy from the baby.

Variation/Tips
- You may need to give a sharp tap or two on the bottom of the turned-over cup to release the flour.
- A food scale is useful for weighing the removed flour.
- If you want a group game, use a cereal bowl instead of a cup and place a small pacifier instead of cereal on top of the mound. Players take turns spooning away a minimum of a tablespoon of flour on their turn. Avoid making the pacifier fall on your turn.
- As a bonus penalty on the group game version, the player who causes the pacifier to fall has to reach in and retrieve the pacifier using only their mouth.

ONION PEELING

An appealing present is revealed under layers of gift wrap.

When
before/after baby is born

How
To prepare, you'll need a prize in a small box. Wrap the prize in gift wrap, then wrap it again and again until it's wrapped in at least ten layers. As you're wrapping the gift, randomly tape a lottery ticket or dollar bill on every other layer, these are consolation prizes.

To play, everybody stands or sits in a circle. They pass the gift around while you play music. Randomly stop the music, whoever has the gift when the music stops gets to remove one layer of wrap (those who come across the ticket or dollar bill get to keep it). Continue until a player gets to the present.

Variation/Tips
❑ Play a song with frequent occurrences of the word "baby," guests pass the present only when they hear "baby" sung in the song.

❑ Try to use different colored or patterned gift wrap to make the layers easier to distinguish. Or alternate between two different colors of wrapping paper.

❑ Variation for a large guest list: eliminate players who get a consolation prize from the circle. This way, those who don't get a small prize still have a chance at the big prize.

❑ For a more elaborate variation: attach a line of instructions on each layer. The player passes the gift to the person described who then gets to remove the next layer and reads the next set of instructions. For example, "You can see in your hands a wonderful prize, so pass this to the one with the darkest eyes." See the Appendix for a full set of rhyming instructions, or create your own. The last person to unwrap the layer that reveals the prize gets to keep it!

PACKING FOR THE HOSPITAL

Predict what will go in mom's hospital bag.

When
before baby is born

How
Ask father-to-be to join in as the hospital trip packer (if he's not available, have mom select a substitute). Give your packer a small overnight tote, tell him he has two minutes to go into mom's bedroom to pack 20 items that he thinks his pregnant partner will need for her trip to the hospital to deliver her baby.

While he packs, everybody, including mom, makes a list of 20 things they think might get packed during those two minutes. Then have dad bring the bag before the group and go through the items one by one. (You might even ask for a brief explanation on any unusual items.) Whoever has the most matches on their list wins.

Variation/Tips
❑ If substituting someone for dad, make sure mom's comfortable with their foray into the bedroom before playing.
❑ Provide pen and paper to everyone before sending dad packing.
❑ If it's too imposing to access mom's bedroom, play this variation. Each player draws a tic-tac-toe square on their piece of paper. In each square, players write down items they think mom will pack for the hospital trip. Meanwhile, mom makes a list of at least 20 items she'd pack. Then as mom reads off her list, guests cross out the matching item (if any) on their squares. Whoever gets a horizontal, vertical, or diagonal tic-tac-toe first wins. Or, to make the game last longer, require people to cover the entire square.

PASS THE PACIFIER

Work together to pacify the baby.

When
before/after baby is born

How
Form two teams, each team stands in a line. Give everyone a plastic straw to hold in their mouth. Give the head of each line one baby pacifier to hold with their straw (hook the pacifier ring on the straw). The leader must pass the pacifier onto the next person on their team, who plucks the pacifier with their straw and passes it down the line. First team to finish the relay passes with flying colors!

Variation/Tips
- Try cutting the straw in half to make the game easier to play.
- If a player drops the pacifier, they may use their hands to hook it back onto their straw and continue playing.
- Pacify the losing team with a rematch if desired.

PIN DOWN THE DUE DATE

Creative predictions for the stork delivery.

When

before baby is born

How

Print out a calendar page for the month that the baby is expected. Circle the due date. Post this page on a wall at eye level.

Give each player a sticker (it can be of a baby item, a star, anything simple) and have them write their name on it. Start the playful predictors five feet from the calendar. One at a time, blindfolded players have to place a sticker on the calendar, trying to get as close to the due date as possible. Whoever lands the due date wins.

Variation/Tips

❑ Save the calendar. If baby arrives on a date other than the original prediction, check the calendar to see if a guest landed on the correct date. Send or give the player a prize.

❑ Create a large one week calendar with times on each of the seven days. Give guests smaller stickers to try to land the correct date and time.

❑ The simplest variation of this numbers game is to have guests write down their prediction of the baby's birth date and time, along with their name and contact information, on a pad of paper. After the baby is born, a prize is due to the person who came closest.

❑ If the baby's delivery date is already scheduled and people know the date, try this instead: guess what the baby's weight will be upon delivery. Write a range of weights along a line on a piece of paper and proceed with play.

❑ Other variations on the pin-the wall theme: draw a picture of a baby that you pin up to the wall. Give guests lip stickers, their goal is to successfully "kiss" the baby on the forehead.

POP THE NEWS

Host a big blow-out to announce baby news.

When
before/after baby is born

How
Write information (announcing the baby's sex, name and/or delivery date) on small slips of paper and fold. Blow up a bunch of pink and blue balloons (so that there's enough for everyone attending) and insert a folded paper into each balloon with some confetti, tie with ribbon.

At the appropriate time, the party people pick the balloon they think represents the baby's sex (or pick any balloon of their choosing if the sex is already known). Then everybody has a blast popping their balloon to get the facts.

Variation/Tips

❑ A variation of the big bang: on a sheet of paper, write down the selected baby name and other baby names that were even remotely considered. Cut out all the names. Stick a name into each balloon, inflate and tie with ribbon. Place the balloons all over the area where you are having the shower. Balloon busters try to find the one balloon that has the chosen name in it, they have to bust the balloon by sitting on it and reading it aloud for mom's verification. The one who finds the correct baby name wins with a bang.

❑ Yet another way to play: give each balloon a tag with a funny fortune or phrase related to pregnancy or babies. Only one balloon has the winning phrase, "You're having a baby!" Let everyone pop a balloon and read their phrase aloud. Bust out a prize to the person who finds the winning phrase.

PREGNANT PAUSE

A race to swell up with pride.

When
before/after baby is born

How
Blow up at least ten balloons (they don't have to be fully inflated). This is a contest to see who can tuck the most balloons under their shirt and in their pants at once. Call up volunteers to take turns trying to balloon up.

Whoever gets the most balloons stuffed into their clothing wins.

Variation/Tips
❑   Take pictures of your pregnant players for laughs.

SCRIBBLES

Use childish handwriting to scrawl out victory.

When
before/after baby is born

How
Give everybody a pen and paper. To play, all players have to do is print their first and last name in 15 seconds. There's one rule, however, the signatories must use their non-dominant hand; in other words, right-handed folk have to use their left hand and vice versa.

The most legible John Handcock, as judged by the group, is your winning hand.

Variation/Tips
❏ Another way to play: scribblers write their name with a pen held in their foot. Use markers since they are easy to hold between one's toes and don't require much pressure to leave a mark on the page. Lay down newspaper underneath the paper to protect against ink bleed-through and errant marks.

SOMETHING'S IN THE OVEN

See what's taking shape in the kitchen.

When
before/after baby is born

How
Just a little prep-work is needed to set-up this game. Purchase a set of inexpensive cookie-cutters. Pick out ones that are not easily discernable and/or unusual, pick a couple of obvious ones too. Select at least 6 shapes, up to 12. Use these cutters to trace their outlines on cardboard and carefully cut out the shape. Write a unique number on each cut-out and spread them out on a large cookie sheet.

Pass out pieces of paper and pen to your cookie club. After scrutinizing each "cookie," they write what they believe each shape is supposed to be. When everybody's finished cooking up their best guesses, hold up each cookie in numerical order and reveal what it really is (or what it's supposed to be anyway). Your smart cookie is the one with the most cut-outs correctly identified.

Variation/Tips
- Instead of having guests crowd around a cookie sheet, you can pass the cut-outs around so that everybody gets a good look.
- Place the cut-outs in a cookie jar and let guests blindly pick a cut-out to decorate (with crayons) based on what they think the shape is. Then all the players try to guess what each cut-out is.
- You can award the cookie cutter set or a package of cookies to the winner of the game.

STACK THE DECK

How high can you go on diapers?

When
before/after baby is born

How
Have at least 70 disposable diapers on hand. Challenge willing contestants to see who can build the tallest stack of diapers. Have players go in turns so the diapers can be reused. Record the number of diapers stacked or the height of each tower.

The diaper tower must stand for at least a second in order for the diaper count to be official (in other words, if the tower falls as the 36th diaper is placed on, then the tower is recorded at 35 diapers tall).

At the end of the evening, pile on the praise for your champion diaper stacker.

Variation/Tips
❑ You may want to specify that diapers have to be stacked flat, no standing them on their sides for greater height.
❑ If you're having a coed shower, this game will especially appeal. It also provides nice picture taking opportunities.
❑ Remind stackers that these diapers will be commissioned later for actual use on the baby, so be careful in handling, and no unfolding them.

TOSS THE BOOTIE

Blurt out a bumper crop of baby bounty to avoid getting the boot.

When
before/after baby is born

How
You'll need a pair of baby booties. Stuff a sock or paper towel into them so they'll have some weight, tie the two together at the laces.

The group stands in a small circle. First player given the bootie has to name an item a baby needs, like milk, then toss it to anyone in the circle. The next person to catch it names another item, such as a diaper, and tosses it again and so on. Players cannot name something that someone else has already said. If they do, they get booted from the circle. If they hesitate longer than 3 seconds to say a baby item or if the item has nothing to do with a baby, that player is also out. Game continues until there's only one player left. Bestow the baby booties on your winner.

Variation/Tips
- If you don't have any booties handy, substitute a teddy bear, or a baby rattle, etc.
- Examples of things a baby needs: blanket, sipper cup, ear syringe, thermometer, etc. You can impose a rule that limits "things" to physical items only or let players get creative (cuddling, burping).
- Make it a rule that a player cannot toss the bootie to the same person who threw them the bootie on the previous turn—unless there are only two players left.
- This non-competitive variation has guests tossing a ball of yarn instead of a bootie. Players have to hold onto their end of the yarn before tossing the yarn ball to another player. Players who are "out" do not leave the circle, they just can't accept any more yarn. Play continues until the yarn runs out, you'll have this fascinating little web connecting the toss-ups together.

Everything's ducky if water runs off your duck's back.

When
before/after baby is born

How
You'll need a large roll of tin foil, a baby tub full of water, and a generous collection of pennies to play. Give each player a two foot long piece of tin foil. They have five minutes to construct a ducky for the baby tub. Do not tell your water fowl inventors what's in store for their duckling before they're finished building them.

Have everybody put all their ducks in a row—in the water that is. One at a time, a player places pennies on his/her duck's back to see how many pennies their duck can hold. The ducky that holds the most pennies without sinking or losing its pennies wins its maker bragging rights.

Variation/Tips
❑ If a duck isn't constructed in a way that easily holds pennies, or pennies keep sliding off the sitting duck's back, make a small indent in the duck to hold the pennies or disqualify the lame duck.

❑ If you don't have a baby tub, any bucket, sink or bathtub can substitute. Test each duck's sea legs one at a time.

❑ This variation requires an investment in as many rubber ducks as you have attendees. With a waterproof marker, mark one duck on the bottom with a star. Place all the ducks in a baby tub of water. To play, tell guests to each pull a duck. Whoever has a star on the bottom of their duck wins a prize. You may choose to let guests keep their ducks as a party favor.

❑ A generous alternative to the above variation is to number every duck, and assign a prize/favor to each number. Whatever number a guest gets on their duck, they get the corresponding prize. Everybody gets something and there's no crying fowl.

WATER WAIT

An ice-breaking race to break your water.

When
before/after baby is born

How
Prep work: you'll need an ice cube tray and green peas (fresh or frozen) or small buttons. Fill the tray a third full with water and freeze. Put one (or two, for twins) pod or button in each ice cube and fill the tray with water and freeze again. Make one "baby" per guest.

Give each arriving guest a cube in a plastic cup with their name on it and congratulate them on their bundle of joy. Your expectant parents guess what time their baby will be delivered (completely free of the ice) by writing their prediction on their cup. Parents have to labor to keep an eye on their water baby. When the little one breaks the ice, write the actual delivery time on the cup. The predicted delivery time that comes closest to the actual time wins.

Variation/Tips
☐ Tape paper to each cup to provide a writing surface if needed.
☐ An alternative: guests race to see who can deliver their baby first. Distribute the babies in plastic cups to everyone at the same time. It has to be a natural birth: parents can't touch the ice cube directly or put anything in the cup itself to induce delivery. First one to completely melt their ice cube and deliver the sweet pea (or button) wins.
☐ Instead of peas or buttons, substitute miniature plastic babies (you can find them at a craft or party store).
☐ This version lasts longer: you'll need a small plastic egg for each guest. Put a marble in each egg (to weigh it down) and put each egg inside a small paper cup. Fill the cups with water (leaving half an inch for expansion) and freeze. Play like the alternative described above.

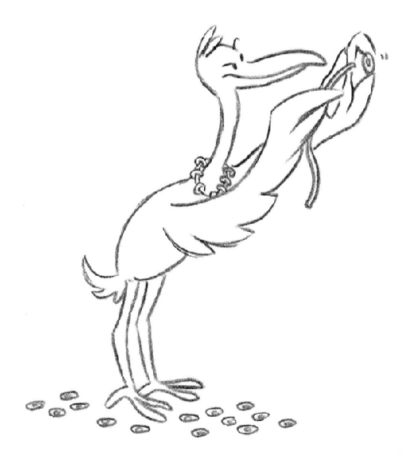

CRAFT GAMES

BIB WEAR

Conceive terrific threads for the toddler.

When
before/after baby is born

How
This artful apparel activity is more manageable with a smaller guest list. You'll need to supply plain white bibs (one for each attendee) and a variety of non-toxic fabric paints.

Give each designer a bib to decorate for the baby. Mom may elect to award a prize to the person who delivers the prettiest bib, most creative bib, etc.

Variation/Tips
☐ Make one ahead of time to give your guests some ideas.
☐ To cut down on costs, create three teams of designers to work on three bibs.
☐ Impose a time limit of 10 minutes to prevent guests from losing focus on their creations.
☐ Or instead of decorating bibs, try simple picture frames.
☐ A popular variation is to provide each guest a 5X5 or 3X3 inch square of light-colored fabric with the invitation so that they may decorate it at their leisure. Collect the squares at the shower and display for guests to see. Afterwards, a sewing whiz can make a quilt out of the squares for mom.
☐ Another alternative: purchase a stuffed animal made of canvas or some other pen-friendly fabric. Guests can autograph the plush toy and write a brief message to the baby on it. The stuffed animal is then given to mom as a keepsake.

BABY CAKES

A cute and competitive cake walk.

When
before/after baby is born

How
Make a two-tiered diaper cake for mom, then players guess the number of diapers that went into making it.

You'll need disposable diapers (number varies depending on how big or small a cake you want, start with 45). For the first tier, tightly roll a diaper into a neat cylinder. Wrap another diaper around the cylinder and another around that. Keep building onto the diapers evenly to create your bottom layer of cake (while keeping count of the diapers used). The more diapers you use, the larger the diameter of your bottom layer. After using up about 28 diapers, tie a wide ribbon around the circumference to prevent unraveling. Make the top layer several inches smaller in diameter than the bottom layer and stack. "Frost" the cake with a baby blanket or colored cellophane, ribbons, other necessities such as a rattle, teething ring, pacifier, bibs, etc.

Keep a sign-up sheet next to the cake for guests to write their name and the number of diapers in the cake. Guest who comes closest to the actual number wins. After the game, mom takes the cake!

Variation/Tips
- Try making a three- or four- tiered cake. Insert a thin dowel in the center, through the layers, to keep tiers in place.
- This is a piece of cake if you start with a roll of toilet paper as your center and wrap the diapers around the roll for each layer.
- Instead of diapers, use rolled wash cloths or socks to create a little cupcake instead.
- After everybody's seen the diaper cake, cover it and let guests compete to recall all the baby things that were on the cake.

BABY TALK

Molding baby necessities from clay.

When
before/after baby is born

How
You can solicit just five players for the first part of this game or invite everyone from the start. Give those playing a small jar of modeling clay to construct an item a baby needs, such as a baby carriage, teething ring, cradle, etc. Without telling anyone what they're making, the sculptors have three minutes to construct it.

After everybody has finished their creation, line up all the creations on a counter or table and number them. Now everybody, including the sculptors, has to write down what they think each item is.

When all clay mates have cast their lots, ask each artist to take turns explaining their custom creation. Award one point for each correct answer, person who gets the most points wins.

Variation/Tips
□ Instead of having players make something of their own choosing, create "playing cards" of various baby items and have players draw a card that tells them what item they have to create.
□ Use fresh clay for best results.
□ For an immature twist on this game, artists may speak only in baby talk about their creation.

BOTTLE YOUR FEELINGS

Encapsulating love for the baby.

When
before/after baby is born

How
You'll need an empty wine bottle with its label removed, a cork to go in it, and one-inch wide strips of paper (cut a regular piece of white paper lengthwise).

Ask guests to hit the bottle with a message or advice to the baby that the child can read when he or she turns 16. Bottle up these messages and put a cork in it. Present to the baby on his/her 16th birthday.

Variation/Tips
- ❑ To better seal the bottle, light a candle and drip some wax around the seal.
- ❑ Use a straw to help push the messages through the bottleneck.
- ❑ If 16 years is too long to wait, make the bottle a one-year time-capsule instead. Memory makers write about the shower or other current events in their lives. Mom opens the bottle on the baby's first birthday.
- ❑ Send a message in a bottle to the baby's sibling. Instead of guests writing notes to the baby, they write notes to the sibling. The bottle can be presented to the child for opening when the baby is delivered.

CONCEIVING BABIES

Behind the back ways of making a baby.

When
before/after baby is born

How
Have all your players stand in a line. Give each a blank piece of paper to hold behind their back. They have a maximum of four minutes to fold, rip, and tear the paper to create a shape that looks like a baby. Whoever tears out the most believable baby wins.

Once a player finishes making the outline of a baby, they are allowed to display their baby in front of them. Have mom and/or the group judge the best looking babe when everyone is done.

Variation/Tips
❑ It's more fun to have everyone stand in a circle facing each other during this game. The faces people make as they're trying to create a baby behind their back can be quite amusing.

❑ Admonish players that they cannot peek at their handiwork until they're done! If a competitor is caught looking at their piece of paper to check their work, that player must stop and deliver their work-in-progress as is.

❑ Do not impose a time-limit for more refined results. If players are taking too long to finish, declare a one-minute warning and wrap up the game.

IT'S ALL RELATIVE

Deliver a baby spud with relative features.

When
before/after baby is born

How
This requires some prep work, but the payoff is hilarious. To prepare, you'll need photographs of mom and dad as well as their relatives such as their parents, aunts and uncles, brothers and sisters. You'll only be using the facial features from the picture, so make sure the face is clearly visible. Portraits are ideal. Make one color copy of each face, enlarging them to almost life-size if possible. Cut out the eyes (keep the bridge between the eyes so they stay together), nose, and mouth of each of the faces. Put all the eyes in one pile, the noses in another, etc.

You'll need two big baking potatoes and a stapler. When you're ready to play, call up a volunteer to randomly select a pair of eyes. Staple the eyes to the potato (turn it length wise so that the "face" is oriented up and down). Select another guest to close his eyes and randomly pick a nose. Staple the nose to the potato under the eyes. Finally, have someone select a mouth and attach. Tada, present this baby to the expecting parents. Make another spud baby if time and enthusiasm allows.

Variation/Tips
❑ Slice some potato off the bottom so the face has a flat surface to stand for display. Or, instead of potatoes, use paper plates.
❑ The eyes, noses, and mouths should be similar in size for best results. Enlarge or reduce on the copier as needed.
❑ Forget the random drawing, let players pick facial features of their choosing to build the baby's face.
❑ Instead of applying the facial features to a potato, arrange them directly on top of an enlarged color copy of mom's (or dad's) face.

116

More than a spoonful of joy with cereal.

When
before/after baby is born

How
Give each competitor a generous bowl of cereal (the kind shaped like an "O") and a handful of string licorice. The object of this cereal commotion is to string cereal onto the licorice and make as many cereal bracelets, necklaces, anklets, belts, etc. as the player can wear.

The person wearing the most cereal by the end of a five minute period wins!

Variation/Tips
- If the contest is too close to call, use a food scale to determine the winner.
- Don't have any cereal on hand? Elbow or wagon wheel shaped dried pasta makes a great substitute.
- Let people pair up for this variation. Each team's assignment is to create a new toy (like a car, hanging mobile, or rattle). Provide crafty constructors with edible materials. Anything that makes a suitable kiddy snack will do as raw material: graham crackers, string licorice, cereal, candy, etc. Give them 10 minutes to construct something. Have each team take turns explaining how their toy works and what it teaches if it's an educational toy. Take a vote among guests for their favorite toy.
- Another way to play: provide a bunch of crafting odds and ends such as scraps of fabric and ribbon, paper cups, straws, cotton balls or pads, cotton swabs, craft sticks, tape, tissue, string, whatever is on hand. Guests create a baby out of the supplied materials. Then mom judges the baby she thinks is the cutest, most looks like mom, or is the funniest, etc.

MATERNITY LINE

Guests conceive their own line of maternity wear.

When
before baby is born

How
Divide the attendees into groups of three. Give each group two rolls of toilet paper and a balloon. The groupies have to dress a member of their team with the toilet paper—without using anything else such as tape or pins to hold it together. The outfitters have six minutes to piece the maternity material together and it must incorporate the balloon to simulate a pregnant tummy. Mom gets to judge the best outfit.

Variation/Tips
❏ An alternative to maternity clothes is to create baby clothes instead. (Lend some stuffed animals as clothing models.)
❏ Give your designers a roll of plain white paper and a roll of colored or patterned paper for more creativity.
❏ A great twist on the classic game: have guests take the amount of toilet paper they normally use when going to the bathroom. They now have three minutes to construct something for the baby. Provide tape.
❏ The success of this elaborate variation depends on the enthusiasm of your guests. Invite couples to participate in a baby fashion show in the invitation. They are to bring all the props they need to dress their partner up as a baby. Put on a "fashion show" and hand out awards to the cutest, most realistic, funniest, and ugliest baby.

Folding giggles and good cheer into a diaper.

When
before/after baby is born

How
Distribute a newborn diaper and bright-colored marker to each person. Each participant writes a peppy phrase of encouragement or a ticklish tease on the outside of their doting diaper. These diaper dispatches will hopefully put a smile on mom's face during those dreaded midnight changings. To get creative juices flowing, here's the straight poop on some phrases that could go on the diaper:

"Only a couple years until potty training!"
"Great oaks from little acorns grow."
"Oops, I did it again!"
"Thanks, mom."
"Danger: Poop Factory."
"Wash me."

Collect all the diapers and present them to mom.

Variation/Tips
❏ For more creative results, send the diaper to guests with the invitation and instructions to write a message. The diapers are then collected at the shower. Let mom read the phrases back to the gathering who then try to guess who wrote what.
❏ This variation is more sentimental. Before the party, ask guests to bring a brief poem or reading about motherhood. If your guests are linguistically gifted, encourage attendees to write their own poems, which can be sentimental or funny or both. Have everyone take turns reading what they've brought for mom and the group to enjoy. Collect all the quotes and poems and present as keepsakes for mom.

MY BABY DOLL

Everybody takes a paternity test after this baby making session.

When
before/after baby is born

How
Have everyone sit in a circle facing inward and give each person three pieces of newspaper. (The host or a volunteer will sit out to run the game.) With their eyes closed, each person has to labor for two minutes to make a three-dimensional baby out of their allotment of paper.

When two minutes are up, everybody sets their baby down in front of them and turns away so they're facing out of the circle. (If a player finishes early, the player turns away and waits.) No peeking! Tape a number to each baby and quickly make a record of the person who delivered each baby. Then mix up the babies, placing someone else's baby behind every player. At the word "go," everybody turns around and has two minutes to locate their baby doll.

Read off your birth records to see which parent has reunited with the baby they birthed.

Variation/Tips
- To ensure nobody peeks, you might want to hand out blindfolds made from strips of fabric.
- Prepare strips of paper with unique numbers (or baby names) on them before the game. Then tape a strip to each baby's wrist or ankle to help quickly ID every baby.
- Take pictures of everyone and their babies for souvenirs.
- This variation uses chewing gum. Give every player a big chunk of gum. Their goal is to chew it until it's pliable, then form the gum into a baby on the gum wrapper. Mom-to-be judges the best formed baby.

APPENDIX

SWADDLING A BABY

Use these instructions on how to swaddle a baby for the It's a Wrap game variation:

1. Lay a receiving blanket on a flat surface and turn it so that it's a diamond shape. Fold down the top corner about 6 inches.
2. Place your baby on his back with his head on the fold.
3. Pull the corner near your baby's left hand across his body, and tuck the leading edge under his back on the right side under the right arm.
4. Pull the bottom corner up under your baby's chin.
5. Bring the loose corner over your baby's right arm and tuck it under the back on his left side. That's it!

TAKING NAMES VARIATION

Here's a list of some modern names and the name they're derived from for playing the etymology variation of the Taking Names game.

Andrew	Andreas	Judy	Yehudit
Anthony	Antonios	Mary	Miriam
Catherine	Hekateros	Kevin	comen gein
Christopher	Christos	Robert	hrod beraht
Emily	Emil	Stephanie	Stephanos
Isabel	Elizabeth	Sydney	Saint Denis
Jason	Iasthai	Tom	Te'oma
Jennifer	Guinevere	Timothy	timan theos
John	Ioannes		

MORE FAMILY NAMES

Additional animal groupings you can use for the Family Names game:

Creature	Grouping	Creature	Grouping
bison	herd	mares	stud
boar	singular/sounder	mules	barren/rake/span
chickens	brood/flock/peep	penguins	colony/muster/parcel
doves	dule	pigs	herd/litter
elks	gang	quails	bevy/covey
finches	charm	rhinos	crash
flies	business	sparrows	host
goats	flock/herd/trip	turkeys	rafter
greyhounds	brace/leash	wolves	herd/pack/rout
hawks	cast/flight	worms	clew

WISDOM TEETH QUESTIONS

Additional questions you can use for the Wisdom Teeth game:

What are the signs that a baby is teething?
What supplies do I need to bathe a newborn?
How do you choose a good pre-school?
What's a subtle way to breast-feed a baby in public?
What do I do for diaper rash?
What's a positive way to discipline a child?
Describe a game I can play with my baby?
How do I ease the pain for a teething baby?
What are healthy finger foods for kids?
How can I get baby to sleep?
How do I burp a baby?
When should I burp a baby?

WHO'S YOUR MOMMA GAME SHEET

Use this sample to create your own game sheet, answer key below.

Draw a line matching the mom with its baby:

cat	baby
cow	calf
dog	calf
whale	caterpillar
pigeon	cub
horse	chick
fish	duckling
butterfly	foal
beaver	fry
insect	gosling
goose	joey
duck	kit
kangaroo	kitten
monkey	kitten
bear	larvae
chicken	puppy
seal	pup
fox	squab

Answers to Who's Your Momma quiz:

cat/kitten	insect/larvae
cow/calf	goose/gosling
dog/puppy	duck/duckling
whale/calf	kangaroo/joey
pigeon/squab	monkey/baby
horse/foal	bear/cub
fish/fry	chicken/chick
butterfly/caterpillar	seal/pup
beaver/kitten	fox/kit

ONION PEELING VARIATION

This version of the Onion Peeling game uses the rhyme below. Pre-game prep: copy then cut out each verse, wrap a gift in 12 layers of wrap, but on each layer tape a verse on it. When a recipient unwraps a layer, this reveals a new verse to read aloud. This verse instructs him or her to pass the gift to another person. The next person unwraps, reads the new verse, passes, and so on.

There are only 11 verses below because the last layer you wrap on the gift has no verse—the first player starts by unwrapping a layer to reveal and read a verse. Make sure you wrap the gift in the order given below (from top to bottom). To see how this will read during the game, read the poem from the bottom up.

❏ Time's up and the wrapping is quite thin! The nearest person wearing a watch gets in!
❏ Relax and don't be nervous, give to the person who lives the farthest.
❏ And not to leave anybody out, pass this to the person who is shortest beyond a doubt.
❏ Not surprised to see another layer more? Give this to the person closest to the door.
❏ Here's another chance just to be fair, give to the person with the longest hair.
❏ Who here wears the longest shoe? The gift now passes to you!
❏ Learning foreign languages is much easier when young, pass to the first person who can greet you in another tongue.
❏ Somebody else's turn at this prize is due, now give to someone wearing some blue.
❏ Look around for the person with the biggest grin, a chance to remove a layer they win.
❏ Hey good-looking, pass this to someone who does great cooking!
❏ You can see in your hands a wonderful prize, so pass this to the one with the darkest eyes.

You can also use a story like the sample below for a Minding Your Fruits and Vegetables game variation.

To the new parents,
We're PLUM crazy over your bundle of joy! If she's a girl, she might have CHERRY red lips or a RADISH blush to her cheeks, either way, may she be one cute TOMATO. If he's a boy, may he always be the APPLE of your eye and a PEACH with the ladies. When the stork finally TURNIPS with your little SPOUT, your friends and family will be RAISIN the roof.

If you CARROT all about your baby, LETTUCE know you will check your baby's diaper regularly, because it PEAS a lot! When people TURNIP their noses and cry sour GRAPES, you know it's time for a changing. And try not to SQUASH the little RASPBERRIES in that dirty diaper, it'll raise a big stink.

Make no BEANS about it, OLIVE us want to give parenting advice, but it's up to you to CHERRY-pick what works for you. Never BEET your child. Remain cool as a CUCUMBER by always counting to ten, after all, the baby is a human BEAN too. No one ever said RAISIN a little ONION would be easy, it's even natural to feel a bit MELON-choly at first. Try to nap the same time as the baby, otherwise lack of sleep will make any MANGO crazy.

Lastly, teach good manners to your child, like saying PEAS and thank you. Try not to let your kid's CORN-ball antics drive you BANANAS. Eventually, your offspring will PEAR up with the love of his or her life and get a great job that comes with a big CELERY too! Now, ORANGE you excited to have this baby? Go forth ENDIVE into parenthood!

PRIZE IDEAS

Offering even the most modest of prizes has a way of motivating shower attendees to play with enthusiasm. Below are some suggestions for rewarding your gracious players. Pick and choose to your taste from the list or let it inspire more gifts.

- ❏ Candy/chocolates/cookies
- ❏ Candle
- ❏ Picture frame/photo album
- ❏ Potpourri
- ❏ Cookbook/gift book
- ❏ Plush animal/toy
- ❏ Inexpensive jewelry/make-up/hair accessories
- ❏ Candy jewelry (necklace, ring pop, gum lipstick, etc.)
- ❏ Pretty note cards
- ❏ A nice/funny pen
- ❏ Bottle of dishwashing liquid/gloves
- ❏ Soap/bubble bath
- ❏ Bottle of lotion
- ❏ An address book/notepad
- ❏ Movie tickets/movie rental gift card
- ❏ One crisp new dollar bill/lottery ticket
- ❏ A bottle of bubbles
- ❏ Corkscrew/bottle of wine
- ❏ A package of coffee or tea or cocoa
- ❏ Current month's cooking/lifestyle magazine
- ❏ Small flowering/evergreen plant/flower seeds
- ❏ Any props used in the game

GAME INDEX

A HOT SHOWER
For a gals-only gathering, games your chick clique will love:

Baby Cakes, 112

Bean Counters, 10

Belly Ache, 37

Bottle Your Feelings, 114

Chaperone, 39

Doctor's Orders, 16

Food Groups, 91

Household Goods, 46

Maternity Line, 118

Mom's Pride & Joy, 47

Mommy's Purse, 50

Piece of Cake, 74

Quadruplets, 23

Safe to Eat, 27

Something's in the Oven, 105

Stork Delivery, 54

Sweet Expectations, 79

Ugly Duckling, 108

Whispering Sweet Nothings, 82

Wisdom Teeth, 57

DADDY'S IN THE SHOWER
While all the games in this book are fun for gals *and* guys (think coed or couples shower), these are even better when dad wants to play:

Bundle Up, 13

Conceiving Babies, 115

Ice Cream Scooper, 95

It's a Wrap, 20

Kidding Around, 63

Lending a Hand, 96

Meeting of the Minds, 65

Mom's Pride & Joy, 47

Name Calling, 68

Packing for the Hospital, 99

Scribbles, 104

Spooning the Pudding, 30

Stack the Deck, 106

Stork Delivery, 54

Wee Gulps, 32

Wisdom Teeth, 57

DISTANT SHOWERS
Whether showering at a restaurant or office or showering an out-of-town mom, these games are easily transported or mailed. (If mailing, seal each game answer in an envelope to be opened after play.) Check out the suggestions for A Sudden Shower too.

Childproof, 40
Count Off, 42
The Funnies, 61
Multilingual Baby, 67
Parts of a Whole, 72
Piece of Cake, 74

Popularity Contest, 77
Rhyme and Reason, 78
Stats, 52
Stork Delivery, 54
Who's Your Momma, 56
Word to the Wise, 83

A SUDDEN SHOWER

No advance prep or special props (just pencil and paper or less) needed for these instant party games.

Artistic Savant, 9
Bedtime Story, 36
Conceiving Babies, 115
Copycat, 86
Crib Sheets, 43
Dating, 87
The Family Name, 61
Good Neighbors, 92
Hen Party, 94
Kidding Around, 63
Lending a Hand, 96

Maternity Leave, 64
Meeting of the Minds, 65
Mommy's Purse, 50
My Baby Doll, 120
Name Calling, 68
News Flash, 69
Popularity Contest, 77
Safe to Eat, 27
Scribbles, 104
We're in the Money, 81
Who's Your Momma, 56

A GENTLE SHOWER

See the Craft Games for non-competitive activities. Skip singling anyone out for a prize so everybody comes out a winner with these:

Baby Sitting, 60
Dating, 87
Diaper Duty, 45
Good Neighbors, 92
Kidding Around, 63
Lending a Hand, 96

Minding Your Fruits &
   Vegetables, 66
News Flash, 69
Stork Delivery, 54
Whispering Sweet Nothings, 82
Wisdom Teeth, 57